For all the twin families – past, present and future – who experience joy, delight and awe but also hard work, concern and responsibility on their special twin adventure.

CONTENTS

PARENTING TWINS

S o you are pregnant with twins or already have twins! How surprised were you or even shocked at the news? Did you think that you knew nothing about twins? If you were in Nigeria that would have been different: Nigerians have the largest number of twin births in the world. But if you were in Asia, say Japan, then you would also be surprised as they have the lowest number of twin births. So what would you like to know about twins to help you on your twin journey??

Let's start with the most basic: You already know that twins occur in at least two different ways. One way involves one egg, fertilised by one sperm which splits sometime after fertilization, thus producing what are commonly called identical twins. The other pattern involves two eggs, each fertilised by two separate sperm, which eventually produce fraternal twins. Fraternal twins may be of the same gender or different genders. In either case, the woman eventually gives birth to two babies, more or less at the same time.

MYTHS ABOUT TWINS

Twins occur in all cultures although they are more prevalent in some than others. This fact has given rise to a wide variety of myths about twins. One of the most famous myths about twins appears in the Old Testament in the Bible. In Genesis, we find the story of Esau and Jacob, twin sons of Isaac and Rebekkah. When Rebekkah's curse of barrenness was lifted, she became pregnant with twins who struggled together in her womb. When Rebekkah enquired how she could live with this, she was reassured with the following:

> Two nations are in thy womb
> And two peoples shall be separated from thy bowels:
> And the one people shall be stronger than the other people:
> And the elder shall serve the y0unger. (Genesis 25:23-4)

In due course Rebekkah gave birth to male fraternal twins. The first born, a red-headed hairy chap, was named Esau; his brother, clutching his brother's heel at birth, was named Jacob. As the boys grew up, Esau became a hunter and Jacob a herdsman. The elder was portrayed as a physical man and his brother a student of the law. Differences thus established, the storyteller continues with an account of how Esau, at a time of great hunger, sold his birth right for some lentils to his younger brother Jacob. Jacob, aided by his mother, deceives his father by preparing a special meal and donning goat's skins on his arm to be hairy like his brother. Not only does Jacob rob his brother of his birth right, but he also steals the blessing of his father which was intended by birth for the eldest son, Esau.

The Jacob and Esau story involves two ideas in twins' mythology. The first is the idea of *unity in difference,* that is, their destinies are bound up with the fact that they are twins (unity), but also with the fact that they are non-identical (difference). The second is *the foundational myth* which rests on the fact that as they are non-identical which necessitates one twin deceiving the father at the expense of the other twin.

At the personal level, twins may be presented as intense rivals even before birth. Other Biblical twins, Pharex and Zarah, are described as being even more vigorous *in vitro*, each struggling to emerge first. Birth order is depicted as having extensive consequences and parents of twins are seen as favouring one twin at the expense of the other, often due to birth order.

The story of Esau and Jacob is a classic foundation myth. Here the Genesis quotation indicates that two nations are to be born and Jacob is himself said to have had twelve sons, the founders of the tribes of Israel, each born with a twin sister!

But probably the most well-known foundation myth in Western culture is the story of the founders of Rome, Romulus and Remus. The twin sons of Mars and Rhea Silva were thrown into the Tiber River by their grandfather's brother, Amulius. Instead of drowning, they were washed ashore where they were suckled by a she-wolf and reared by a shepherd. When they grew up, they avenged themselves (on Amulius) and subsequently founded the city of Rome in 753BC on the spot where they were rescued. In a later quarrel, Romulus killed his twin brother Remus. So this twinship obviously resulted in conflict and destruction rather than in harmony!

Greek mythology is full of stories of twin births and twin divinities. As in other cultures, the Greek myths explores twinship as it involves *double paternity*. One twin is viewed as the child of a human father and the other has a divine father. The most famous twins in Greek mythology are the Dioscuri, Castor and Polydeuces, even better known by their Latin names, Castor and Pollux. There are various versions of this myth: in one, the god Zeus unites with the mortal Leda and produces two heroic boys; or in another version Leda and Zeus have two sets of twins, Castor and Clytemnestra, and Pollux and Helen (later of Troy), sometimes thought of as quadruplets. In the double paternity version, Leda is depicted as being impregnated both by Zeus in the form of a swan and by her human husband King Tyndareus. Thus Zeus fathers Pollux and Helen, and Tyndareus fathers Castor and Clytemnestra.

Similar variations occur in the subsequent accounts of the lives and fate of the Dioscuri. These emphasize their heroic status as fighters, leaders in battle, great horsemen, and rescuers. However while these accounts describe the Dioscuri as very close, some tales make distinctions as in the Esau and Jacob case. Thus Castor is portrayed as warlike, aggressive and rash, whereas Pollux is more passive and more domestic. But these versions do emphasize the inseparability of the Dioscuri. When Castor the mortal is killed, Pollux the immortal begs Zeus to share his brother's fate. Zeus consents and the united twins share time in either heaven or Hades, or on earth and on Mount Olympus. In their honour, Zeus creates the constellation Gemini (the Heavenly Twins). In general, the Greek deity myths of the Dioscuri have the twins worshipped as divine.

Similar patterns of divinity occur in other mythologies, including in Indo-Iranian mythology. While the Asvin twin brothers' paternity is somewhat unclear, unlike the rivalrous behaviour of Jacob and Esau or the extreme fratricide of Romulus and Remus, these twins are portrayed as inseparable companions, as deeply loving twins, even compared to a happily married couple!

In North and South America, there are numerous pairs of divine male twins. These twins are thought of as personifications of the Sun and the Moon: the elder twin is the Sun and he, the clever one, continuously restores his brother, the foolish, the lazy brother, on a monthly basis as the Moon. In some tribes the divine pair introduce a variety of techniques considered to be useful to mankind. There are many examples such as the Navajo and the Zuni who believe that the Sun fathered divine twins who perform enormous feats to reduce a multitude of dangerous forces opposing mankind.

It is quite evident, even from this small sample, that twins are conceptualised in myths both as positive and negative, harmonious and rivalrous, happy and unhappy, divine and human. They play a role in foundation myths and in double paternity or birthing myths. Looking worldwide, twin myths contain stories about (twin) gods who are deified men or women. Some even try to provide some answers to life's unanswerable questions. Some twin myths try to legitimize societies.

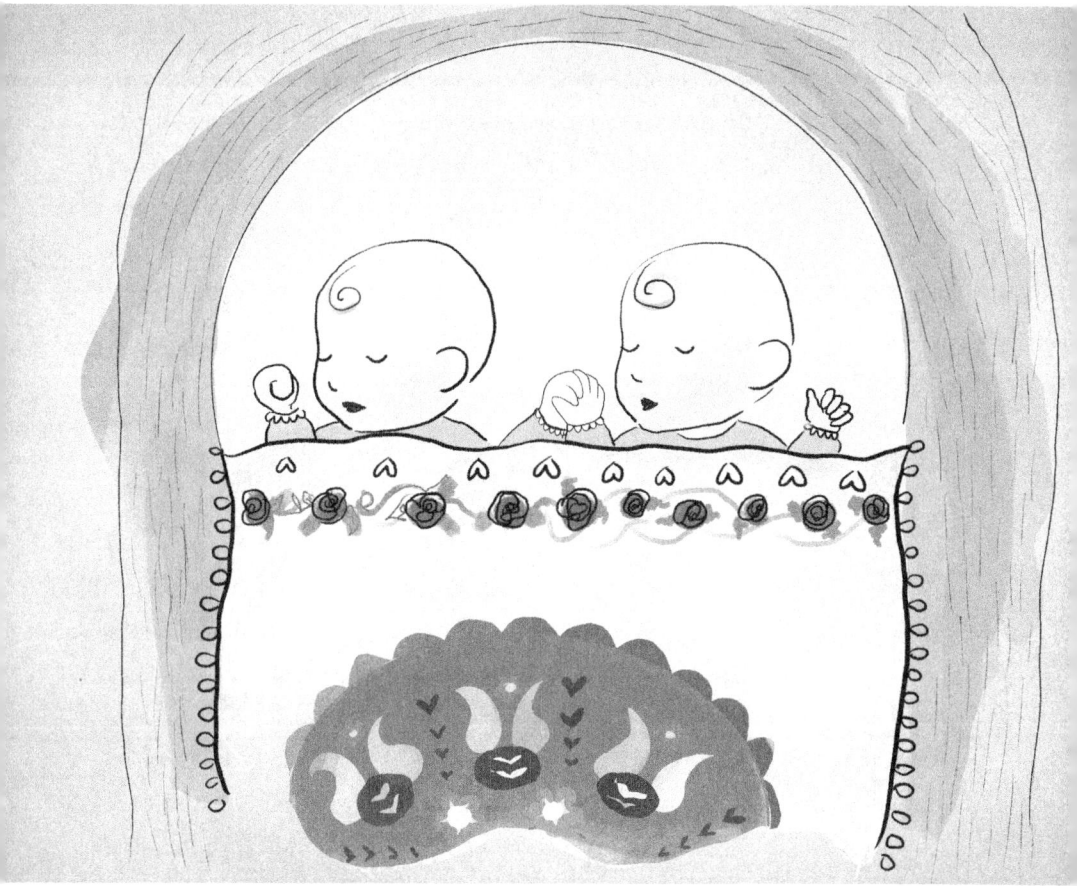

Twins have provided an endless source of fascination for storytellers and writers for centuries.

As twins appear in a wide variety of cultures, twins are viewed as the ideal vehicle of exploring the nature of identity, be it personal, social or moral. The search for identity appeared alongside using twins to illustrate a wide range of differences. Initially the overwhelming focus of attention was the comic potential of mistaken identity using identical twins. But then writers began to explore proposed contrasts, such as good versus bad, like versus unlike.

Literature

Shakespeare was himself the father of fraternal twins, Hamnet and Judith. Twins figure in at least two of his plays. In *Twelfth Night, or What you will*, fraternal twins Viola and Sebastian so resemble each other that, were it not for their clothing, they could not be told apart. When circumstances place Viola in a strange country after a shipwreck, she puts on male clothing, adopts a new name and goes to serve as a page. The play progresses with each twin looking for the other and climaxes after episodes of mistaken identity, leading one twin to marry in place of the other. The twins are described as having the same face, the same voice, the same habits. So even opposite sex twins are thought of as being fundamentally similar, which was common in Shakespeare's time.

In his second play, *The Comedy of Errors*, Shakespeare has two sets of twins fastened to two strong ships' masts which saved them during storms at sea. The two sets of twins were born in the same inn to two different mothers, one the wife of a wealthy merchant while the other wife was very poor. The wealthy merchant buys the second set of twins to act as servants for his children. These male twins are described as being exactly alike in face and person. After the shipwreck, many comical blunders occur as of course two sets of identical twins appear on stage. Mistaken identity abounds in a real 'comedy of errors'. So twins are used by Shakespeare as entertainment.

After Shakespeare, the increasing use of twins illustrates the growing concern with issues of identity. In Mark Twain's works, Twain (or Samuel Clements) deals mainly with **issues of identity**. He often concentrates on alternative selves people can have, but also looks at the question of how to differentiate one person from another, how we tell people apart. For example, in *The Prince and the Pauper*, the prince is mistaken for the pauper and the pauper for the prince. Both men are portrayed as pseudo—twins.

6

Authors then focused on the process of **doubling** as characters searched for his or her own identity. The idea here is that we are all made up of two parts, often complementary: such as partners or enemies, good or evil, innocent or criminal. Twins in this literature often fall into the good/evil category as in the *Man in the Iron Mask* story where the king has his twin brother imprisoned and masked. Or in *The Corsican Brothers* story (both by Dumas) the brothers are united both in life and in death by an essentially loving bond. In Bruce Chatwin's *On the Black Hill*, twin farming brothers spend most of their lives together secluded in rural Wales.

Another topic writers turn to is the area of horror and science fiction, both in print and in films. Often macabre stories are developed, such as the horror of doubleness is explored for a Siamese twin pair who are joined front (one's chest) to rear (the other's back.)

Children's literature and television

Stories about twins abound in children's literature. They are often humorous and full of fun. Perhaps the oldest from our standpoint is *Alice's Adventures in Wonderland* where funny identical twins, Tweedledum and Tweedledee, are hard to tell apart. This is obviously not the problem in the **Topsy and Tim's** books where these twin children are used so that boy/girl issues can be looked at. Equally sometimes they are just used as same-aged kids experiencing some situation in slightly different ways. In the States, the *Bobbsey Twins*, another boy/girl pair, were used to solve mysteries and share adventures.

What happens when single-sex children are used? Of course we would expect a lot of confusion. Take the *Sweet Valley Twins* series. 'As far as looks went, it was virtually impossible to tell them apart, from their long blond hair and blue-green eyes to the dimple each girl showed when she smiles.' But one could tell the girls apart by their personalities, stemming partially from their birth order. One twin was born four minutes before the other and she acts as big sister. These twins are used to represent tensions between different aspects of personality. They are also considered 'special': 'being twins made them as close as any two people could be', but in another book, 'they hardly ever agreed on anything.' So not so special!

Television programmes for children (of all ages) also express themes about twins and twin relationships. In the Australian soap *Neighbours*, female twins are originally introduced by showing them as witnesses to a crime. The twins are subsequently in hiding because of course finding two females who look alike is easier for the villains then finding only one. But as the situation changes, the twins are portrayed as quite different in characteristics, even if they look very similar. In an American series **Beverly Hills 90210** boy /girl teenage twins are featured and like Topsy and Tim the twins are used as vehicles for exploring a variety of problems faced by each twin. Usually the problems are specific to their gender.

Twins in Films

Films which are not especially for children often focus on a good/evil split between twin siblings. Here the evil brother/sister tries to stamp out his good brother/sister, but often good triumphs over evil. Thus the stereotypes about twins are reinforced in the media while the films illustrate and explore themes of personal and social identity.

The single and largest group of 'twin' films emerged from the American studio system in the 1940s. With varying degrees of subtlety and inventiveness, the twin films used a variety of combinations of moral and psychological differences in the guise of good and evil. Then twins were used to illustrate personal and social dilemmas, to explore possible responses to important social problems.

The theme of mistaken identity and its consequences is central to the enormously successful Disney family film, *The Parent Trap*, remade in 1999. Identical twin girls are separated when very young because their parents get divorced; one girl goes to live with their mother, the other with their father. When they meet by accident at a summer camp, it becomes clear that neither knows of the other twin's existence. Startled to see someone looking exactly like themselves, the girls slowly become friends during the summer. They hatch a plot to re-unite their parents by switching places. Each girl goes to live with the other parent, thus assuming her sister's role. It is only with time, it seems, that each parent realises that he or she has 'the other' girl twin. The parents meet to 'exchange' children and in true Disney fashion decide to become re-united. The happy ending thus involves not only the re-united parents, but also reuniting the girls who are allowed once more to become 'real' twins. In this way, the film strongly and affirms the unity of twins.

In sharp contrast with this comedy of mistaken identity is the treatment of twinship in David Cronenberg's film, *Dead Ringers* where identical twin boys grow up to become eminent gynaecologists. As young twins, we see both boys equally interested in science and medicine but at the same time they are shown with marked personality differences. In the present, the same situation applies: one twin is extrovert, the other introvert; one is the initiator of their research work, the other carries out that research; one is a 'ladies' man, the other is much more reserved. The problem arises when the introvert falls for one of his patients, but is unable to act upon his feelings. It is therefore the extrovert brother who originally seduces the woman *for* his brother. Throughout the film, each brother continues to absorb the feelings and actions of the other. As one brother becomes dependent on drugs but is subsequently able to conquer his dependence, his brother takes over and, in turn, becomes drug dependent. In other words, throughout their lives these men search for their own identities, but in the end - an end which leads to both of their deaths - this proves impossible. The film ends with the bizarre and disturbing image of the brothers acting out their separation as if in reality they were Siamese twins. In fact, their own mental image of themselves involves the story of the well-known Siamese twins, Eng and Chang, who lived physically joined but distinct lives with their own families, but who died in fact within two to three hours of each other.

While there are many other examples of twins in film, one other film cleverly exploits audience pre-conceptions about twins, at one level subverting such pre-conceptions while affirming them at another. Ivan Reitman's *Twins* refreshingly departs from those possibilities of twinship which dominated the past-World War II films: double image, mistaken identity, a bodily split between good and evil. In *Twins* we are presented with brothers who are the product of a test tube sperm combination of many distinguished fathers and the egg(s) from one mother. Separated at birth, one twin played by Arnold Schwarzenegger has brains, brawn, looks - and an environment filled with everything possible to encourage mental and physical growth. The other twin ends up in an orphanage, scraggly, homely, in trouble, with no prospects. When the brothers meet at the instigation of the luckier twin, the other, played by Danny DeVito, looks at Schwarzenegger in total disbelief. He is saying (and the audience is thinking), you must be joking - we can't be twins because we do not look anything alike, let alone look identical. After all, we *know* that twins always look alike. Yes, twins can be fraternal, but this is ridiculous! In other words, the film challenges our preconceived ideas about twins, and it is this challenge that makes the film so successful and so funny and, one must add, a great hit for many twins themselves.

The Press

Let's not concern ourselves with those newspaper or journal articles which use pictures and stories of twins just to establish exactly how similar twins are. Nor will we be bothered with the sensational press, with articles, for example, which deal with twins as freaks, whatever our definition of freak may be. Here I wish only to consider the broadsheet press and materials found in those magazines or journals which not only deal with human interest stories but have some practical implications as well.

We can easily characterise the press' coverage of twins by applying the following five broad divisions.

The first category involves *famous twins* and *famous parents of twins*. Articles often appear about twins who are well known or are celebrities, especially about those twins who are famous because they are employed in the same field of activity. So in the film world, we have film directors and producers such as the Boulting brothers; in the sports world, the Gulliksen twins, Tim and Tom; as agony aunts, Dear Abby (Abigail van Buren) and 'Ann Landers'; in the criminal world, the Kray brothers; in the arts, the Singh twins. Sometimes, we are made vividly aware of the public success of one twin, although the other twin's life is more private, such as in the case of the boxer Henry Cooper and his brother, and the racing driver Mario Andreotti and his brother, or of a 'lone twin', such as Elvis Presley. Parents of twins may also be singled out, such as Judy Finnigan of Richard and Judy fame, George Clooney, Julia Roberts, James Purefoy, Michael Buerk the newsreader. And the famous tennis superstar Roger Federer has two sets of twins. Maybe the most famous, however, is Lady Thatcher, former prime minister of Great Britain.

The second type of image in the press stresses the *unusual nature* of being a twin. Most often mentioned here is the supposed telepathy between twins or indeed their psychic affinity. Stories are often told of how one twin, many miles from their twin, experiences similar pains as their twin brother breaks his arm or twin sister goes into labour. Or there are reports about the murder of one twin and the article explains how the surviving twin copes. There are even reports about the murders of both twins. (April 1997)

The next group of articles can be described as articles about **twin birth** itself and the subsequent **parenting of twins.** The first subdivision looks at discussions about the possibilities and benefits and consequences of fertility treatment, especially IVF. Medical ethics may be explored: if more than three foetuses are successfully implanted, does or should the couple have the choice of aborting any of them? The second subdivision involves a wide range of articles on the parenting of twins. They could easily be titled as follows: a) So, you're going to have twins! b) How to help yourself during a twin pregnancy! c) How to bring up and manage two babies! d) How I survived twins and lived to tell the tale; and e) Sources of help.

The fourth division involves articles on **what it is like to be a twin.** The material here is almost limitless, but may range from articles on how it really feels 'to be half of a pair' to advice to teenage twins on surviving adolescence in the presence of your twin. These articles tend either to stress the fun elements of being a twin, as in 'playing the twin game', or to tackle seriously the twin situation as experienced by other twins. More recently, this category has included articles on the position and feelings of the 'lone twin', that is, of the twin who loses a twin through death at whatever age.

The final section could be entitled twins in **science and nature.** This often revolves around questions dealing with intelligence and the measurement of intelligence. Journalists attempting to examine the nature of intelligence - Is it determined by inheritance? Is the key factor the environment? Are some races or social classes more intelligent that others? - usually quote material relating to twins. Quite often twins separated either at birth or sometime thereafter are used in these discussions. These twins fascinate not only journalists most interested in scientific reporting but those who wish to tell stories of what we shall here label coincidence: for example, how separated twins Barbara and Daphne choose the same clothes, have three babies in the same gender order, fall down and injure themselves at the same age. Articles discuss the general role of genetics in all of our lives, often using twins to illustrate whatever point they wish to make. [In the next section, we shall examine more deeply these questions of science and nature.]

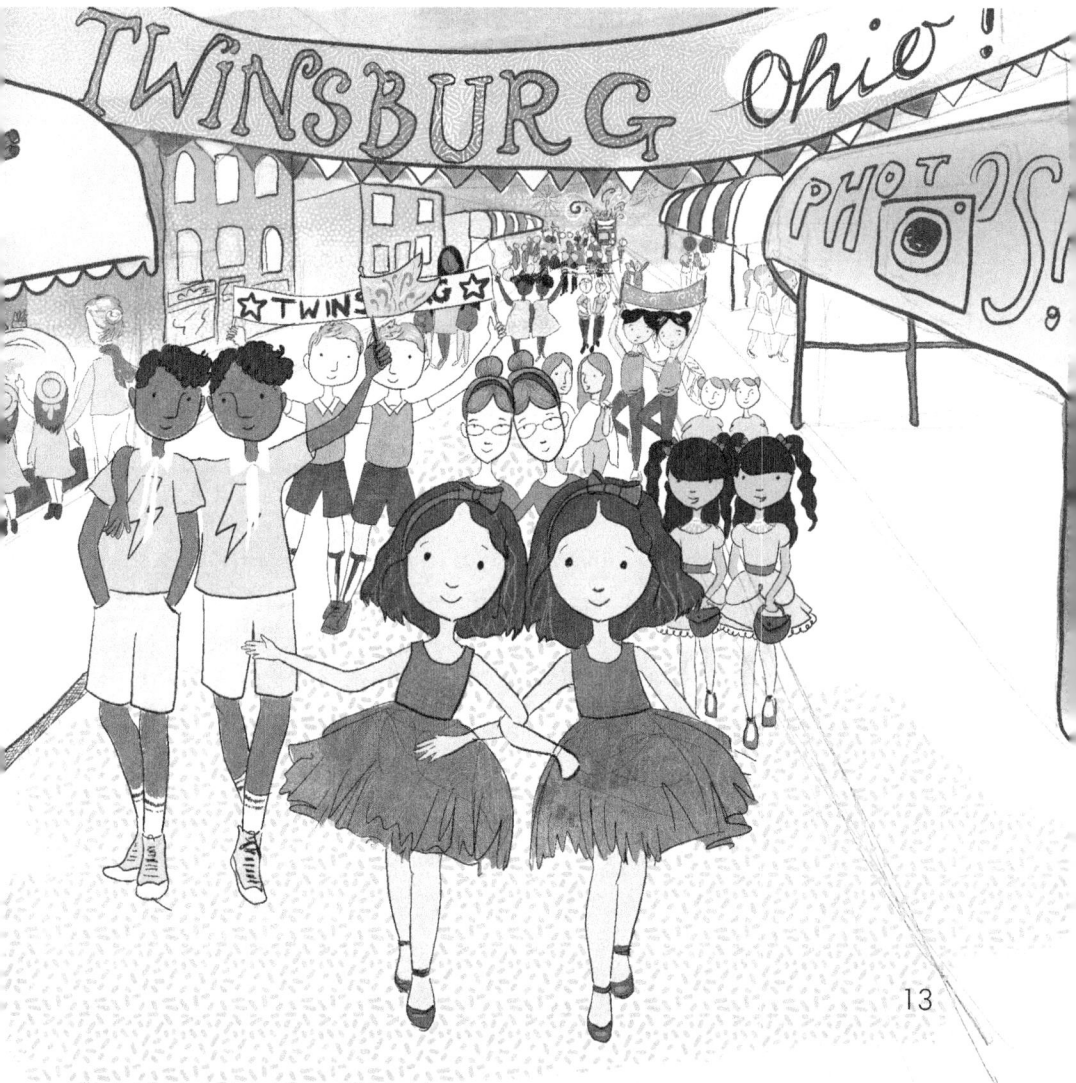

NATURE/NURTURE

Maybe you have been asked to participate in some research using twins, or maybe you will be. Or maybe you have heard about the nature versus nurture arguments about twins. So how does this affect you? How did this argument or division actually come about?

In the ancient medical world, the birth of twins was treated as a unique and specific phenomenon; subsequently medical researchers also viewed twins mostly from an obstetrical point of view. But in the second half of the nineteenth century the study of twins took a different path with the work of Sir Frances Galton, a cousin of Charles Darwin. So instead of twins being a biological or obstetrical curiosity, they were used as a research tool. Galton hoped to be able to distinguish the effects of birth from the circumstances experienced throughout life. And here is where the serious study of twins begins.

In order to study twins, the researchers had to distinguish the two types of twins. Twins are either identical (monozygotic) or fraternal (dizygotic). Twins are monozygotic if a single fertilised egg divides sometime between the first and fourteenth day after conception; twins are dizygotic when two separate eggs are fertilised by two separate sperm. This is significant because identical twins share the same set of genes whereas fraternal twins are no more alike than any other siblings, that is, on average they share 50% of their genes, [although some authors have claimed that same-sex dizygotic twins share genes in the range of 25 to 75%]. In other words, the heredity factor for monozygotic twins is identical or, at the very least, more similar than for dizygotic twins whose shared heredity is more variable. Therefore, since the heredity or genetic factors are the same/similar for monozygotic twins and different for dizygotic twins, the **twin research method** is based on the proposition that one can distinguish the effects of heredity and environment by comparing these two types of twins.

This classic twin method, as we shall see, assumes that while heredity differs for the two types of twins, the influences of the environment are the same or equal for the two types. Thus any differences between identical twins are due to environmental or at least non-genetic functions. The corollary to this is that the degree to which identical twins resemble each other (in comparison with fraternal twins) mirrors the impact of the hereditary contribution to any particular characteristic.

Within this general perspective, twins are used to try and discover which traits and/or diseases are genetically determined and to what extent genetics determines the particular condition. Let us take some examples. If one monozygotic twin has, for the sake of the argument, cerebral palsy or heart disease or six fingers, what are the chances that his or her same sex twin has or will have the same condition? What role, if any, does the environment play in the determination or formation of any particular disease or condition? This research model, known as the twin clinical method, can be further divided into four cases:

1) Both twins are affected in the same environment E.g., both get measles

2) Only one twin affected in the same environment. E.g. poisoning of one

3) Both twins affected in different environments. This is the case of hereditary diseases.

4) Only one twin affected in different environments. Very useful to study the influence of the environment on the disease.

In addition to examining twins genetically in relation to health, medical researchers also study twin *pregnancies*. Research here is concerned with the health both of the mother and the babies as distinct from managing a singleton birth. For example, what are the medical hazards of a twin pregnancy, at what stage (and with what consequences) is a twin pregnancy diagnosed, how does the obstetrician manage a diagnosed twin pregnancy, what are the adequate stages of intrauterine growth for twin one and twin two, what risks does each of the twins face, how is the actual delivery to be handled, what complications might arise?

Is/was it important for you as parents to know whether your twins are identical or fraternal? Yes and no!! But for research, misdiagnosis can lead to incorrect answers of either genetic or environmental influences. How can we know which type of twin we have? There are several ways of determining twin types. The most effective is by blood typing. There are also ways using finger and palm prints or examining the placentas at birth. More recently – and perhaps most easily - the swabs of cells taken from inside the mouth are the most reliable test. Before this last test, some studies used a physical resemblance questionnaire, sent by mail. Here we have the 'as alike as two peas in a pod' phrase appearing. Other studies asked parents and friends if the twins are frequently mistaken for each other. Or mothers have been asked about the physical similarity between their children and/or do strangers mix them up.

Interestingly, identical twins tend to be misclassified as fraternal twins rather than the reverse. Mothers of actual identical twins were cautious in calling them identical, often preferred to call them fraternal, said they were uncertain or even wished them to be fraternal although recognising that there was a good chance that they were identical, or finally, were simply misinformed at birth [that is, they were told that one placenta meant identical twins, two placentas meant fraternal twins which is now known not to be correct] and hence labelled their twins fraternal. Thus, we have a group of twins who are environmentally or socially fraternal and genetically identical.

Equal environments?

Once twin type is established, researchers want to know the role that the environment plays.

Given the fact that there is a variety of conditions which effect prenatal (foetofoetal transfusion syndrome) and postnatal (different birth weighs or co-joined twins) for twins, it would seem clear that there is no such thing as an 'equal' environment, even for identical twins. Perhaps the way around this problem/dilemma is to visualize environments as being more or less similar, rather than the almost impossible-to-verify pattern of equality. The argument then would be that, as a generalization, the environment for identical twins <u>may</u> be more similar than the environment for fraternal twins. Why? On the assumption that monozygotic twins are genetically similar, their similar physical appearance would encourage those in their environment - parents, peers, teachers, acquaintances, etc. - to treat them in a similar fashion, thus reinforcing their similarities.

On the other hand, it has been argued that parents of identical twins, for example, may accentuate whatever slight behavioural differences that occur in their twins and therefore treat their twins *less* equally. Identical twins may respond to their environment and behave differently, accentuating or emphasising differences, especially as each twin attempts with time to create his or her own identity vis-a-vis their twin. Thus the environments of identical twins could either create and encourage *similar* behaviour patterns or emphasise and accentuate *different* behaviour patterns.

As for fraternal twins, their environment would be less similar than for identical twins because they, again as a sweeping generalization, are not only not as similar genetically but are consequently not as similar in looks. Fraternal twins are assumed to be treated quite distinctly *because* of their different appearance. However, following this line of argument, same-sex dizygotic twins who do look alike would be treated alike and would thus develop similar personalities and behaviour patterns (as is argued for identical twins).

The role of the environment involves *time* as a key factor. When actually is the impact of the environment being measured? -- early in the twins' life (presumably by a parent), during the chaotic time of adolescence, in adulthood? Is the study to be a longitudinal one, tracing changes over a considerable period of time? And, equally as important, what factors are being measured and what effects of the environment are being considered? We must ask: measurement for what, testing for what?

Both types of twins share a similar environment, an environment that is significantly determined by the very fact that they are twins. Both are labelled as twins by the environment inside and outside of the home. Both groups are subjected, at different times, either to a contrast or a comparison effect imposed by their 'environments'. Like other siblings, both types of twins face varying environments due to gender differences, position in the family, spacing of children, types of sibling interaction, relationship to parent(s), etc.

Perhaps the bottom line in the above discussion is the nature/ nurture or genetics/ environment controversy which, like a pendulum, has swung over the years. More and more researchers are looking at the *interaction* of genes and environment. Both factors act as determinants of behaviour in a variety of ways. Perhaps within each individual, at different times and at different ages, and in different situations, the interaction or complementarity varies.

PSYCHOLOGY AND PYSCHOANALYSIS

Besides ourselves, who is interested in twins? One group is the psychologists who have utilized twins in many areas of their research. They look at temperament, personality and intelligence or cognition. In general, the conclusion from all of these areas is that there is evidence of the effects of heredity on these different factors. But there seems to be quite a range of hereditable influence: some authors have demonstrated *moderate to large genetic* contributions to many personality dimensions whereas others focus on *moderate* contributions. While twin studies on personality have changed over the years, the research still tends to focus on genetic variations. [section 4]

Twins were first studied in the 1930s by psychoanalysts such as Heinz Hartmann and Hubert Cronin. They found that the very fact of being a twin, regardless of whether the twin was identical or fraternal, significantly affected the personality development of the individual (twin). In other words, through his or her development at the same time. These analysts stress that there are many environmental factors which influence each and every twin's development, starting from the very fact of being born a twin, incorporating differences at birth for each twin, and leading to a process of 'mutual identification' between twins.

During the war years, four sets of twins and one set of triplets were observed in the Hampstead Nursery [England] for a period of up to four years by Dorothy Burlingham and other staff. One of the many important points Burlingham makes is that a twin may adjust and adapt his/her personality, beginning perhaps in the basic competition and rivalry for parental love. Another pattern is a process of copying: if one twin did something that was of interest, the other twin copied him/her, a process sometimes caused by dependency. This 'other-focussed' activity, says Burlingham, caused development to be hindered in the pair of twins.

Burlingham also describes the behaviour of some twins in terms of their acting as a 'well organised team. In other situations, the team effect was the outcome of learning to temper each of their personalities (that is, to adjust and adapt) so that as a consequence, the twin relationship became the closest tie between the two individuals. This need to establish an equilibrium and to have harmonious relations as a resolution to their rivalry, suggests Burlingham, may be vital to understanding twin development.

Individuation

Since the writings of these pioneers, [Hartmann, Cronin and Burlingham, among others], psychoanalysts have studied twins from a variety of viewpoints. One area of concentration is the **process of individuation**, a process, it is argued, through which all children must ideally pass if they are to achieve personal autonomy. At first, there are no boundaries between the infant and the rest of the world. Slowly the infant becomes aware that the mother (or some surrogate mother) is not merely an extension of his or herself. Thus he/she little by little separates his/her own self from that of the mother. This process of the development of separation, of differentiation, of disengagement from the mother is called individuation.

The process of individuation is experienced by every child. Is this process different for those children who are not singletons but are in fact twins?? If the answer is yes, then is the process different and what, if any, are the consequences?

In the first place, the relationship with the twin, or the intertwin identification, also begins so early that its origin is complex and complicated. And, what, if any, are the consequences? The twin must, because of the essential and fundamental intertwin Identification, also separate from his/her twin. In other words, the twin must go through a twofold process, separating firstly from the mother and secondly from the twin. Before that, one twin may perceive the other twin as though observing himself in a mirror. Conversely, he is likely to think his own mirror image is his twin. (Leonard, p 308)

In other words, throughout the early years of childhood, the twin may only gradually discover oneself as a separate individual. The intertwin relationship persists because other relationships do not interfere with it and consequently the twins are able to fall back on each other, perhaps with some detrimental effects.

Case studies reported in the literature illustrate the problem of individuation from both mother and twin. In one, the authors suggest that a normal separation-individuation process would be different for twins and would frequently be incomplete because: a) the mother is shared by two children and the mothering itself would not be optimal; b) levels of frustration would be high for twins (as the mother cannot meet each child's individual needs as she would a singleton) and therefore the twins would turn to each other; c) the other twin, rather than the mother, thus becomes the comforter and the loneliness and separation anxiety experienced by singletons would not occur; and d) as the special relationship develops between the twins, the mother may become alienated, thus reinforcing the twins' symbiotic association.

But let's keep in mind here that these psychoanalysts are generalizing from individual case histories of some of their patients. So not to worry on this account!!

Other Themes

Most analysts agree that identity formation, stemming from the individuation process, is complicated and confusing for twins. While they have utilised a variety of terms to classify the twin relationship, they have all

- more or less - described a variety of characteristic problems and difficulties faced by twins. This may stem from the fact that the twins may identify with each other and are mutually interdependent. In other words, there is a lack of personal identity. The two individuals function to a degree as one. Most agree that twins have a special problem in achieving separation and individuation, a problem which may lead to a confusion of ego/self, of self-identity, of an inadequate self-image, and of uncertainty about (ego) boundaries. They see difficulty in differentiating behaviour, thought, and wishes from those of the other twin. Each twin must then develop those traits which enable him/her to become a 'whole' separated person.

These characteristics can be supplemented by several other major themes which run throughout the psychoanalytic literature. Firstly, there is the *rivalry* between twins. Some stress this situation as occurring from birth, a situation which thus conditions attitudes, behaviour, etc. The rivalry is depicted as intense. Related to feelings of rivalry are feelings of *ambivalence* about twinship, a problem seen as being connected with the status or condition of twinship. Ambivalence, of course, is related to this rivalry or perhaps is the other side of the coin in that many twins have very strong, warm feelings towards their twin, towards their companion. We need to remember that analysts are looking at those twins in therapy who are the ones who, for one reason or another, were unable to resolve these feelings satisfactorily.

A related theme running through the literature is twins as a **unit.** The consequences of the twins seeing themselves and being treated as a unit are multiple. One way this occurs is that in adjusting and adopting their personalities to make the unit workable, each individual twin either becomes incomplete without the other twin or becomes two parts of a single whole. The end result of this unity may be painful non-individuation, delayed separation, emotional distress. Moreover, the role(s) that each twin plays within the unit may become structured: some twinships may exhibit very strict divisions of who does what and who possesses which traits, whereas other twinships may exchange patterns of behaviour more easily and at varying intervals. Some twins thus work out their individual identities as part of a unit more or less by polarization.

Equally as important, being seen as a unit is often reflected in feelings of being special, feelings which would thus disappear with the severance of the twin link. Would anyone know or notice me if my twin wasn't present or known, let alone not dressed the same or similarly? Experiencing oneself in the unit as special or even exceptional contributes one way or another to individual development, to forming relationships with others, to uncertain skills in being alone and/or to being 'ordinary'. The elimination of the twin unit may be related to the *anxiety of separation* from one's twin. Separation from the twin, occurring whenever it does happen or had not happened, mobilises what most psychoanalysts see as the most basic anxiety, that is separation anxiety, which may lead to reactions of: denial, anger, mourning and grief.

One of the consequences of separation discussed is that of the need to re-create the twinship in other relationships. Old patterns may drive the twin to find a twin substitute in subsequent, intimate relationships. The twin may assume that other relationships will be or even should be similar to the twin relation, thus resulting in a new fused union where the formation of boundaries was previously learnt. Forming relationships with others may be significantly affected by the initial twin relationship.

It is important to note that psychoanalysts do not seem to be as concerned about the actual genetic nature of twins as are psychologists. In fact, very early on Hartmann and Cronin surmised that just being the member of a twin pair, whether identical or fraternal, had profound effects. Burlingham stressed that twins *per se* went through the same stages of development, in close proximity to each other, seeing their own emotions played out in front of them. Or we have the view expressed that 'twins, be they *identical or fraternal*, are often each other's inseparable companion, their physical and environmental lives parallel and complement each other; they are thus each other's intimate environment, affecting each other in innumerable and subtle ways.' (Karpman,264: italics mine) There is certainly evidence to support the idea that zygosity is not the principal factor in determining the psychological development of individual twins.

Psychiatrists, perhaps more than psychoanalysts or psychotherapists, have also discussed a variety of psychotic problems or psychopathological behaviour(s) discovered in certain sets of twins. While too technical for my purposes to be discussed here, these studies have usually concentrated on identical twins, examining one twin for a particular disorder (e.g., schizophrenia) and seeing whether or not his/her twin exhibits similar malfunction. But in general, I would maintain that while zygosity may be important, it is not the sole source of psychological, let alone other, behaviour.

FAMILY, PARENTS and SIBLINGS

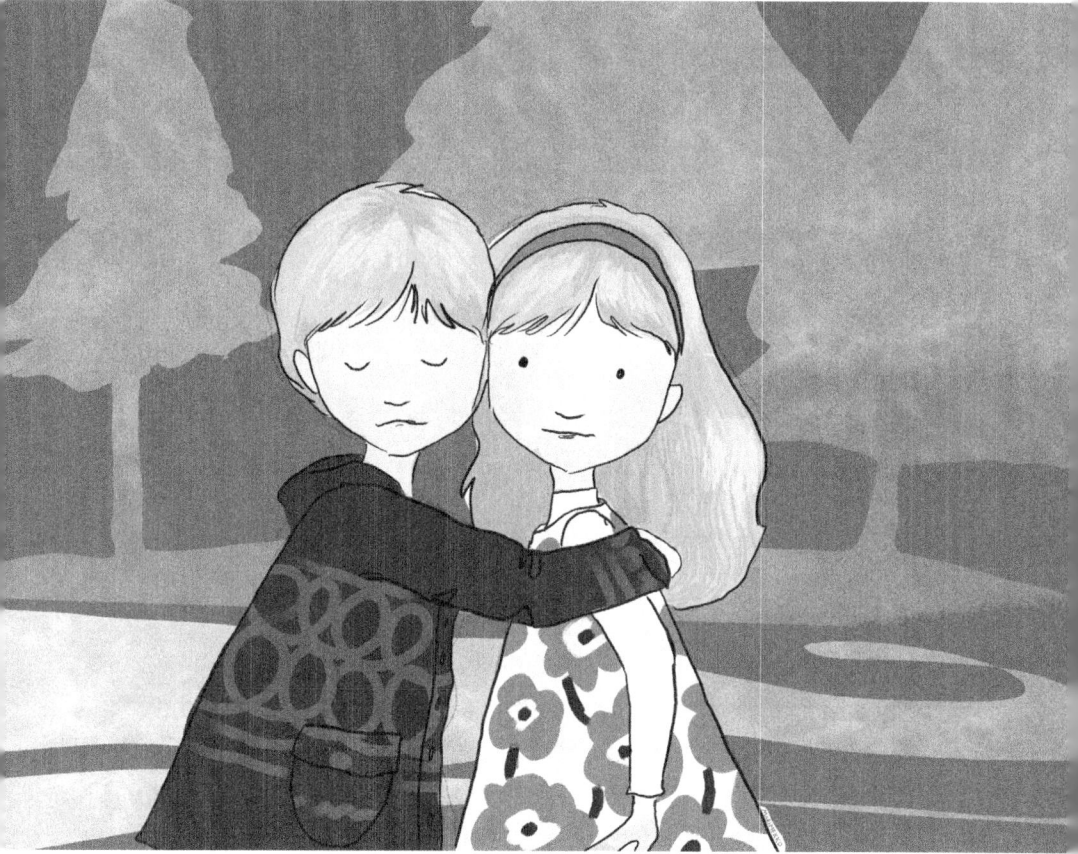

Now you know how twins are viewed by the media, literature, psychotherapists and other specialists. But what are the actual questions you might have concerning either the welfare of your twins, your ability to adapt to a twosome, how your actual family may be affected by the twins, etc. And of course what about the twins themselves! This section looks at similar questions about the considerable number of consequences coming from multiple births. Some of these we may call clearly positive, others much less so. And of course, there are plenty of grey areas here.

Let's start out with the consequences for **the family.**

For most parents, a pregnancy usually results in the eventual birth of one child. A planned pregnancy, whether it encompasses a couple's first, second, third or subsequent child(ren), may often be the outcome of balancing individual and family needs and expectations, and of agreeing on the desirability of a further, let us say, second child as the wished for completion of the family.

The emphasis here is on the second child. Once twins are diagnosed, however, second becomes second *and* third. All types of family configurations may easily be substituted for this example.

The increase in the actual size and the eventual change in the structure of the family because of the very fact of having twins naturally has a variety of repercussions. For many parents of twins, the social disadvantages of having twins begin with the very diagnosis of the twin pregnancy. In the first instance, the diagnosis may have consequences for the pregnancy and for the management of that pregnancy. These may include more frequent visits to the doctor or hospital, more symptoms of pregnancy experienced by the mother, more necessity for managed rest for the mother (for example, hospitalisation before the birth itself, although this practice is becoming increasingly less common), and the necessity for the mother to give up her job earlier than she had expected or had wished. Children already in the family may experience changes in their mother which may be more marked or severe than for a single pregnancy. Physical strain on the mother may be greater, causing her to be more fatigued and less active, less involved with the present child(ren).

Some researchers have even argued that a mother of twins manages the diagnosis of twins with four distinct strategies: seeking information about twins in general, *making room for two*, apprising the risk of having two babies, and engaging in protective behaviours of two foetuses. The second strategy includes grappling with doubts about her ability to cope with two infants simultaneously, relating to the foetal activity of two, attributing personality and gender characteristics to each of the foetuses, as well as dealing with problems of equality with each foetus and with viewing the twins as a unit. (See also mothering dilemmas below.)

If we look at the **economic** factors of twin pregnancies, that is, the costs for neonatal care and costs for care of handicapped children related to twin pregnancies, some studies   indicate that: a) there is an *enormous* increase in the financial cost of multiple pregnancies, and b) these additional costs are highly related to the unfavourable birth weight distribution for twins and higher multiples. [Whether the state (for example, a national health system) or the parents pay these costs is not so moot a point.] The hospitalisation of preterm twin(s) has short-term, as well as conceivably long-term, consequences. Without question, there are extra difficulties for parents of twins who have one or more premature babies. For example, while one premature infant may be in a special baby care unit in the hospital of delivery, the other infant may need to be cared for at home.   Thus the first month(s) of the twins' lives may be in very different environments, requiring quite different skills, energies and material resources from their parents. Moreover, prematurity and/or low birth weight have their own consequences: when two babies are involved - be they in a similar or dissimilar situation or condition - the problems are quite naturally multiplied.

Whether the twins are premature or not, families of twins are more or less immediately faced with purchasing - or securing by any other means - two sets of appropriate clothing and baby equipment, for example, cots, highchairs, car seats, toys, nappies [diapers], and so on. The financial implications, which may be staggering at the beginning, have extensive and indeed may have serious, long-term implications. Thus the family that has planned and budgeted for the first, second, and third child, has not necessarily done the same for the second, third and fourth child, respectively! While it may be relatively easy to beg and/or borrow baby's clothes, converting a small car into a larger car is more difficult, as is moving to larger premises, say, with the same mortgage. The economic consequences may be daunting in the short and long term: holidays (including the perennial problem of what to do during the holidays!), accommodation, travel and transport are all affected by an increase in family size.

The financial implications may be compounded when one examines whether or not the mother returns to work. A study of two hundred families with two month old twins in France confirms that many women (half the women in this sample) did not return to work after the birth of twins whereas the majority would have done so if they had only expected a singleton. The decision to stop working appears to be related for many women to financial problems created by the twin birth, but for others it is a deliberate choice motivated by their desire to raise their children themselves. The decision to return to work is multifaceted, depending on socio-economic status, type of job, partner's income (partner's flexibility?), care available for the children, and the number of children already in the family.

Consequently, twinship significantly affects a variety of chances in life. Let's consider the life chances of the twins themselves. We have already touched on the more limited resources available to the family as a whole and consequently to each twin him/herself. Had the twin been a singleton he/she would presumably have had the benefit of more of the family's financial assets. This applies to smaller matters such as clothing, school trips, leisure pursuits, as well as to larger issues such as travel, holidays, IT equipment, education. In the U.K. and the U.S., it also applies to much larger concerns such as the funding of higher education. As many have found, it is not 'cheaper by the dozen'; substitute 'multiple birth family' for 'dozen' and the outcome is the same. In other words, the family's disposable income has to be shared by more, rather than fewer, people, thus affecting the life chances of the twins as well as of all of the other members of the family, not least with respect to family dynamics in both the medium and longer term.

The more limited financial resources are not the only ones which have to be shared. It is hard not to imagine that any child would benefit from having the exclusive attention from his or her parent for an unspecified period of time and their emotional development may also affected by the number of children. It could be argued that more time is available for each child individually and the relationship of time to child depends on the actual number of children in the family.

Siblings of twins

This brings us to the effects of twinship on the sibling/s already in the family. There is a vast psychological and psychotherapeutic literature on the impact - or more precisely the *dramatic* impact - of the arrival of any child on an older sibling. The concept of sibling rivalry is known not only in the academic world but is also often bandied about by lay people. The effect of the birth of twins on a sibling, however, is much less often discussed in both circles.

Even before the birth of the twins, siblings may be affected. As already mentioned, the mother may be more tired and less active; there may be perinatal birth complications, requiring, for example, bed rest and/or hospitalization. Moreover, as happened in my case, an older child, when boasting of the fact that her mother is going to have twins, may be constantly questioned about the veracity of her statement: surely she is just fantasising about the twins and consequently not telling the truth! [Never before had my daughter encountered such disbelief.] Thus, at the very time when a usually young child is coping with both the external reality and internal fantasies arising from a twin pregnancy, she may be unwittingly denied support by important adult figures in her life.

Once the twins are born, siblings are more or less continually affected. The mother - and usually the father - is very occupied with the exhausting and excessive tasks of caring for two new-born babies - feeding, changing, bathing, stimulating, let alone running a home and a family. The babies may be premature and/or in special baby units, may be fragile, one in hospital and one not. The sheer exhaustion experienced by the mother/parent is hard to categorise, but the sibling(s) no doubt experiences his/her/their parent(s) as at the very least having less time or very little time for them: competition for the parents' attention begins very early on. It has been argued that the child is displaced as a consequence of a single pregnancy but often more so in a twin pregnancy.

Just how long this displacement occurs varies no doubt from family to family, from circumstance to circumstance, but it is a significant displacement. Some families try to ease the displacement by using the sibling/s as mother's little helpers, for example, in feeding or bathing the babies, thus creating the new role not as substitute mother or carer but as secondary/additional/second mother or carer. Some siblings certainly respond positively to their greater responsibilities.

As special praise, let alone attention, is often bestowed on twins from both within and outside the family, the sibling(s) quite naturally may feel displaced at the very least, if not actually rejected and/or ignored. Many a mother of twins has had to gently remind admirers of her twins that the older sibling, who is party to the praise and attention, is an important and special member of the family as well. The attribute of 'specialness', in fact, is the very attribute which the sibling may feel he/she has lost. Instead of being an only child/second daughter/third son, the child has become and is subsequently known as the brother or sister of twins, the focus of only secondary interest and attention. Loss of attention, loss of time, a less energetic parent, lack of one's own space, a change of status - all have consequences for the sibling(s). Siblings may respond by being troublesome, including misbehaving, or by being troubled, exhibiting excessive shyness or being perfectionists so as not to further burden the already burdened parents (Hay).

Child Abuse

Some researchers into the phenomenon of child abuse have hypothesized that the risk of child abuse may be increased in families with twins. This is premised on the knowledge that the risk of child abuse in general increases with family size (for example, larger families are more predisposed to child abuse) and with inadequate spacing of children. Twins obviously fit the latter pattern of 'inadequate spacing', but larger family size may also be a relevant factor. Furthermore, some researchers into child abuse have found a relationship between the prematurity of an infant and subsequent child abuse, as well as a relationship between abuse and an infant's low birth weight. Once again, twins often fall into these two categories.

Does child abuse increase in families of twins? The general conclusion is that the stress of rearing twins is indeed significant. But the simple presence of twins is itself a more critical variable in predicting abuse than the other factors associated with twinness (such as prematurity). That is, the whole family, especially marginally functioning families, are adversely affected.

An unexpected finding from the research is that *siblings* of twins are reported as victims of abuse more frequently than the twins themselves. The simple presence of twins is itself a more critical variable in predicting abuse than the other factors associated with twinness such as prematurity. They affirm that stress is a predisposing factor in child abuse. Parents of twins certainly are confronted with more than their fair share of stress.

Post-natal depression

These considerations predispose one to assume that mothers of twins are more likely to experience post-natal depression than comparable mothers of singletons. Why could this be true? After the birth, there could be more symptoms of stress, and high levels of anxiety and extreme depression compared to mothers of singletons. Other factors could be whether the twins came home at the same time from the hospital and whether one twin had died. In general, the studies conclude that the increased stress, including anxiety and depression evident in mothers of twins, is not specific to twinning per se but is *numerically related to the intense physical and emotional requirements of small babies.*

And a final note, a general point about postnatal depression should be made which applies to both multiple and singleton births. It is often the case that postnatal depression occurs without being confirmed by proper medical diagnosis. Consequently, there may be no medical intervention and/or recognition of the condition. Thus, mothers suffering from postnatal depression may indeed *suffer* from postnatal depression, unaided and untreated by the medical profession. So it is possible that mothers of twins suffer disproportionately more than mothers of singletons, the significant factors being non-diagnosis of post-natal depression due to the possible isolation of the mother in the early weeks and due to the mother's lack of time or energy to visit the doctor.

Bonding

The issue of the bonding between mother and infant is one which is often raised in the context of twinning. The theoretical issue is: can the emotional bond between mother and infant naturally and optimally be established only on a one to one basis? The presumption is that the normal bonding process will consequently be distorted or at least will be more likely to be insecurely completed.

Mothers of twins must bond with two 'new' people more or less at the same time. This process will be difficult because mothers of twins will attempt to meet the needs of two babies, simultaneously. Thus different researchers have concluded quite differently that: 1) the mother of twins more easily or more readily bonds with the heavier or larger twin; 2) the mother bonds with the twin who arrives home first from hospital ; 3) the mother prefers the weaker twin because of her greater concern for this child's health ; and 4) the mother prefers the stronger twin . Gender is only mentioned once when it is argued that males are more 'popular' because they were usually the larger in a pair of boy/girl twins.

Do mothers of twins have difficulties bonding with two infants? Mothers of twins are faced with many 'mothering dilemmas' but many argue that they related warmly to both infants shortly after the birth. Sometimes the preference of the mother for one twin or the other tended to fluctuate over time, while other mothers staunchly rejected the idea that they themselves show preferences for one or the other twin.

Here are some possible circumstances which could influence these mothers in initially failing to bond with their offspring: 1) when the mother has experienced a distressing birth; 2) when physical contact with the babies is delayed; 3) when the babies are very small and premature; 4) when the mother is unable to establish equal contact with each child; 5) where there is insufficient help with feeding or caring for the infants; and 6) when, in spite of all of the maternity staff's efforts, the mother feels both inadequate and demoralised because she feels her management of the infants was inferior to that of the staff. Some conclude that while some mothers report initial deference toward, let us say, the weaker baby, this did not influence long-term attachments between mother and children. By the age of one year, the maternal bond was no longer present with the lighter twin but had switched to a bond with the less competent and more dependent twin.

And a final note, perhaps not so much about difficulties in bonding but more about the mother having to share between and with two babies. Concern for the other twin - say, when feeding, changing, hugging one twin – may mar the pleasure that the mother may derive from caring for one of the twins, that is, the mother is certainly aware of the left-out twin's pain. But perhaps the last word should be left to D.W. Winnicott, the eminent doyen paediatrician, child psychiatrist and psycho-analyst who, when discussing how well the mother is able to give of herself to two babies at once, says in *The Child, the Family and the Outside World*, 'To some extent she must fail, and the mother of twins must be content to do her best, and hope that the children will eventually find advantages that will compensate for this inherent disadvantage of the twin state' (1991, p.139). A rather pessimistic note here!

Mothering Dilemmas

As just stated, mothers of twins face a variety of dilemmas, initially in bonding with their infants but subsequently in relating and caring for two infants. The word 'dilemmas' is used because for many, the handling of the twins is a matter which involves the mother in chronically considering how she can give of herself to the two infants and how can she relate to each child individually. The question of equality is also omnipresent.

Pointing to the ambivalence mothers experience when confronted with multiple births, it has been suggested that mothers oscillate between two patterns. They either view the infants as an indivisible unit, treating them as 'the twins', or, alternatively, they accentuate the behavioural differences of the twins, thus labelling each child differently and consequently treating each child individually. The first approach implies that the twins will be treated 'equally', as a unit. In this case, sometimes the mother is insensitive to the needs of the individual twin. So if one baby cries to be fed, the other is also fed, whether or not he/she is hungry. On the other hand, the process of labelling each child emphasizes or exaggerates the twins' differences. Once labelled, however, it is hard for the mother to see the child in any different light.

There are other dilemmas to be faced. Optimally, the mother has to behave in such a way as to distinguish one twin from the other, while at the same time attempting to treat each child without favour. The differentiating process in the immediate period after birth may involve such processes as the naming of the children such as according to birth order or family resemblance. Or the choosing of specific colours to represent each child (this is my blue boy, this my green one!). At one end along the continuum are those practices of child rearing which reflect very conscious parental choices to differentiate their twins (such as in choice of clothes and toys) and at the other end are practices more compatible with alleviating the mothers' workloads by streamlining routines.

The preceding dilemma is intricately related to another, namely, how to develop the identity of each twin. Is this best accomplished by treating the twins as individuals or by treating them equally or the same? How does one create a happy balance between treating each child as an individual and treating him or her the same as the other child, in order to 'be fair'? Most of the current guides for parents are quite explicit about suggesting that parents should actively differentiate their twins. The proviso, however, is that there are difficulties in implementing these intentions. For example, how does the parent manage a pair of twins, one of whom has some form of special needs?

Parenting

Becoming a parent is not only a physical act. It is a social act. And if the transition to parenthood is a transition to a new social status and to a new network of relationships, then the parents of twins occupy a similar but additional status: they become parents, but they also become parents of an exceptional group of children.

Having been brought up mainly in households with singletons, many parents have no real role models when it comes to relating to their newly acquired 'group'. As we have seen, the media - magazines, newspapers, television - may, for example, help to shape general perceptions about parenthood, but when it comes to twins, they mainly emphasize the 'cutesy' side of twinness, that is, the image of identical twins, the sameness of the children or they emphasize the sinister side of twinship. For example, they find criminal elements in both twins, such as the Kray twins or the more aberrant side of twinship, such as co-joined infant twins. Learning to be a parent of twins may in fact be haphazard. One usually learns to be such a parent as one goes along, without relying on many 'set' rules. Or one exchanges experiences with other parents of twins, many of whom may also be new to the role.

The psychological literature has frequently studied how twins are actually treated by their parents. Much of this work focuses on how one can explain individual differences between the twins, especially identical twins. Studies have confirmed individual differences within identical pairs, explaining that these are due to a complex interaction between 'constitution', differential *parental* attitudes, and the relationship between the twins. For example, some indicate that identical twins are indeed perceived and treated as different children by their parents who, in fact, sometimes exaggerate the twins' physical and behavioural differences evident at birth. That is, parents need to create and even exaggerate differences between their twins so that they may avoid the confusion they feel themselves. Other studies conclude that parents *respond* to rather than create differences between the twins.

One issue not touched on involves parental *preference* or indeed parental *preferences*. Are parents - both mother and father, individually and together - treating the twins more or less equally or are they favouring or labelling or making allowances for one twin as distinct from or at the expense of the other? Does one twin always come first? Is one twin always picked up first? Does one get more attention than the other? Is one labelled more positively and the other more negatively and once done, does this not continue? Does one child become the *mother's* child and the other child the *father's* child? Such parental preferences may be quite devastating for twins who see themselves as being 'endowed' in a similar fashion (in terms of their similar looks and their similar behaviour).

Parents of twins may furthermore be conflicted as to whether to emphasize the twinness of their twins, an act which places both parent and twin in the limelight. Alternatively, should they emphasize the individuality of each twin, thus helping the twin eventually to become an 'individual'? The current emphasis on individuality for multiple birth children is putting even more pressure on parents as they attempt to fulfil the demands of multiples with different schedules, different demands and different levels of development. Their limited resources can be stretched to breaking point. Being the parents of twins is indeed a different experience.

Partners

Another of the serious consequences of multiple births is the possible strain on the relationship between the parent partners. Some studies suggest that mothers are unconcerned during their pregnancy about the emotional stress twins might place on their relationship with their partner. And yet they are unable to get out alone as a couple during the first three months after the birth, a crude index, it is suggested, of lack of quality time together. Other research is even more negative: mothers must negotiate intensified conflicts between their parenting and marital roles and the reduced space in which to meet other personal needs. Furthermore, perceptions of the enormous sudden responsibilities and sense of the inability to cope as a parent, as a spouse and as an individual may often lead to discouragement.

The only counter argument to the probable strain between partners due to the arrival of twins found that the emotional well-being of parents of closely spaced children is more positive for parents of twins than parents of closely spaced children. The respective fathers of twins had pride in the fact that they had produced twins. Notwithstanding this piece of research, few couples who have twins would not but confirm that the twins put various stresses on their relationship. The very fact of having two children at the same time, that is, the hard work involved with having two children, let alone the 'dilemmas' imposed on such couples, produces added strain, strain which is certainly not confined to the immediate period after birth. While an already good relationship has scope to cope with this strain, a poorer one is certainly more limited. Both partners need the emotional support of the other.

Partners may also be confronted with feelings - as well as the reality - of isolation as new parents of twins. After the 'high' of being the centre of attention in hospital, eventually they must return home to a more private environment. Without the aid of an extended family, a fact which is becoming more and more of a pattern in modern post-industrial societies as jobs take couples far from their parental homes, the partners may indeed have to face their new responsibilities all alone, without much familial support.

What about fathers? Above we spoke about depression in mothers, but a state of depression must be raised here as regards fathers. Some work suggests that with the birth of twins fathers experience the loss of their partner, sometimes the loss of their partner to technology (to IVF, for example). If one or both twins are premature, they also feel a loss of the child to the hospital's technology as well as a loss to and an invasion of other people, incorporating the medical world and including in-laws. While all children more or less bring a reduction in parental flexibility, fathers of twins certainly experience this decrease in flexibility and an additional decrease in mobility. Finally, fathers may experience a change in their relationship with their partner because of what they perceive is a loss of equality. Their partner - the twins' mother - may become the dominant person, the person in control of the twins' situation.

A final note here. It is often said that the presence of multiple births in a marriage may contribute to divorce. While there are 'folk' discussions about this, I have no general or specific statistics. We do know, however, that there are a considerable number of single parents raising twins. We also know of teenage mothers raising twins alone. Statistically, however, we do not know if the correlations exist.

WE TWO TOGETHER

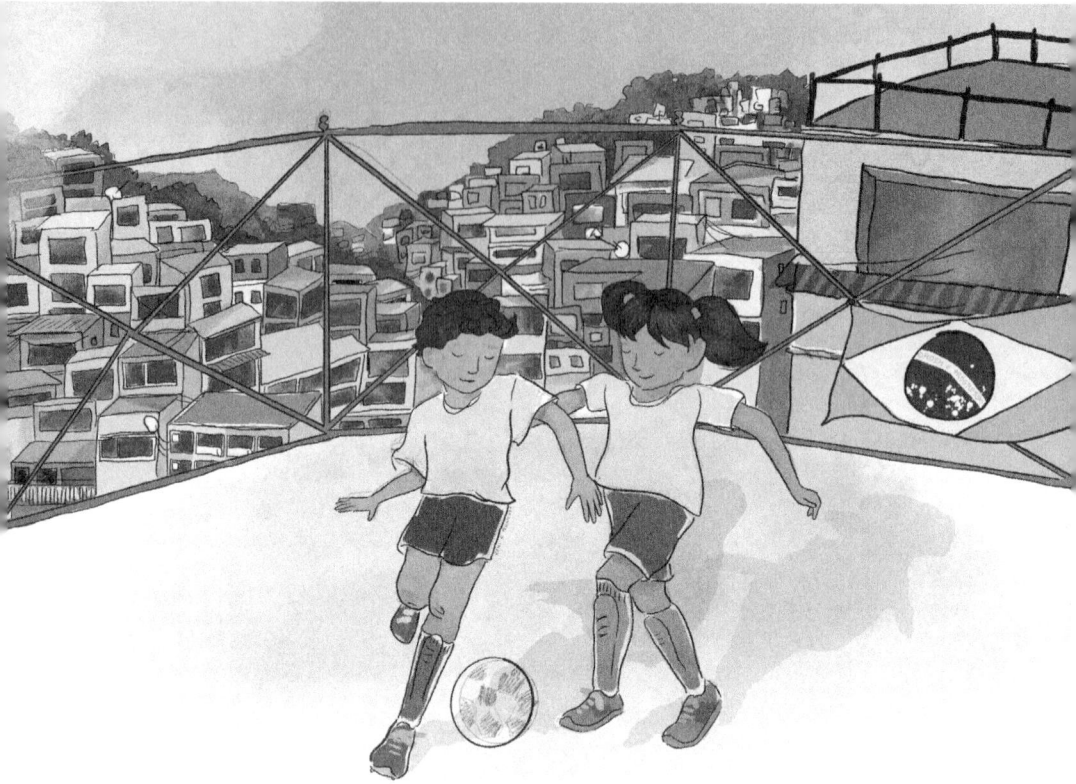

aving considered the social consequences of twinship as they affect the family, parents and siblings of twins, we now turn to some social consequences for the twins themselves. The base line for examining the repercussions of twinship is often comparison with singletons. The result of this comparison is that twins are thought to be variously 'disadvantaged' in relation to singletons because of the very fact that twins come in pairs. Let's first consider some general disadvantages, then move on to language development, followed by the educational system, and conclude with a discussion of arguably the greatest trauma for any twin, the death of the other.

General disadvantages

The argument begins in the social science - as well as the medical – literature that as compared to singletons, twins themselves experience greater stress during gestation, during delivery and during the early perinatal period of their lives. The biological differences appear to indicate that twins' earliest days are marked by potentially more hazardous conditions than singletons. Reassuringly, these initial physical experiences and weaknesses are overcome by the age of eight.

What then are some of the other, nonphysical manifestations of the disadvantages of twinship for the twins themselves? One such disadvantage is the effect of one twin on the other in the form of *peer distraction*. Some maintain that peer distraction is actually an essential feature of twinship which does not automatically disappear with the end of childhood.

Competition between the twins is another factor of twinship which does not appear to end at any set time. It is argued that twinship provides each twin with another person with whom he or she may or can compete, whether the competition always or sometimes -- but usually *not never* -- takes place. Competition may in fact begin in the womb, the very essence of the competition being who comes out first: the 'who arrives first' factor may also be a continuing, even all pervasive, factor in the twins' relationship.

Twin competition expresses itself in numerous and pervasive ways. A few examples in the early years would include competition to acquire food (the best ice cream cone), toys (the biggest fire engine), clothing (the 'coolest' outfit), let alone competing for the attention of adults in the form of, say, crying. As they get older, twins at the Oedipal stage not only compete with their *parent* of the same gender but also compete with their co-twin for the affection of the opposite-sex parent. In fact, the term *rivalry* may be the term more applicable throughout a twinship rather than merely competition.

In the school setting, twins compete not only with other children, but compete with each other (see below). This competition is often reinforced by teachers and other pupils. Both groups, for example, may conclude that a one-point difference between the twins in a test is a significant factor, a factor worthy not only of commenting on but also of actually utilising to taunt one twin at the expense of the other. National testing, with results for GCSE and A-levels or SATs, may often be stormy times in the lives of twins and their families. [One of my colleagues tells the story of twins at an American Ivy League University, both of whom had the highest grade point averages for years. Their marks were separated by .2 or .3 of a point. Consequently, one was known as the successful twin and other as the twin that failed!] In adolescence, the competition may (but not often) take the form of vying not only for friends but also for the very same person. Most siblings compete with each other. Perhaps twin siblings do so at a more heightened level.

In spite of competition or rivalry, twins may create a unique **bond.** The twin bond no doubt varies over time and varies both within and between twin pairs. The extremes of this bonding have taken the form described by Marjorie Wallace between the *Silent Twins* (1986), female twins who in their bonding together dramatically failed to separate from each other, became elective mutes and were eventually committed to Broadmoor (the British asylum for the criminally insane).

But the twin situation could also be more **positive**: twins never need to be lonely. Let us suppose that a twin has misbehaved and the parental way of dealing with this child is to send him/her to his/her respective room. This twin is often 'visited' by their twin or even brought presents, such as food offerings, thus negating the isolation tactics. Or, supposing an outing is planned, is not the one twin to be affected by the behaviour of the other? Furthermore, twins have the possibility of *emotional support* from each other, a feature which has its positive and negative sides. While emotional support may be sustaining or stifling, a same aged child's emotional support may not be as adequate or indeed as mature as emotional support from an adult.

In the last analysis, however, as singletons we have not experienced an omnipresent twin sibling, both from a positive or a negative standpoint.

Language development in twins

The development of language in singletons is a complex process and this statement could equally be applied to the development of language in twins. The fundamental issue seems to centre not on the actual process of acquiring language, a process which many agree follows more or less similar patterns for preschool children, be they singletons or twins. The argument is founded on over fifty years of research which indicates that twins - on average - *may* experience delays in language development when compared with singletons.

Many researchers, when asking the question as to why this may be so, suggest that language delays may be caused by greater prenatal and greater perinatal problems experienced by twins. Is the reason for language delays in twins due primarily to these 'biological' causes? The majority of researchers conclude that this is not the case, although some highlight the increased *risk* factors for twins.

Some argue that the major cause of language delay is that parents of twins simply speak less often to each child separately, let alone to the twins together. This is due to the reduced opportunities for interaction between parent(s) and twin(s) which affects the twins' abilities to experience adult language. As parents are involved in much greater physical demands in caring for two babies, they interact verbally less often. Twins may experience less praise and less approval from their parents, as well as fewer verbal refusals and fewer threats. The thought is that twins are therefore exposed to a decreased quantity of and a lowered quality of speech, but not necessarily actually neglected.

Parents are also implicated in creating or not creating the possibilities for socialising with other children. Parents of twins are accused of introducing their children less frequently to other children. This lack of socialisation reduces the twins' abilities to broaden their social and language skills. Others have concentrated on the increased interaction between the twins themselves. They argue that this produces less of a need for the twins to communicate with others because of the close bond created between them and therefore they are sufficient company for each other.

Some argue that a link between the twins is created to such an extent that they will be less motivated to communicate verbally with others because they already understand each other's gestures and facial expressions. Twins may create a **secret language**, a language unintelligible to others but used by and understood by the twins themselves (known as cryptophasia).

But many others do not believe that twins create a secret language. Twins instead of inventing a secret language enter a competition for adult attention and then adapt a variety of strategies for this role, such as speaking very quickly in order to attract attention away from their co-twin. This process should not be examined in terms of language delay or a secret language, but should rather be considered as adapting language to a different situation (to 'turn taking'), to the twin situation, and as reflecting an efficient use of language, given the situation which involves two same aged children plus an adult.

The jury is still out on which factor - twinship, closely spaced children, social class, parental interaction - is paramount in its impact on language retardation. However, twinship is a contender. Being a twin *per se* may just result in being in an 'impoverished' language learning environment.

Educating Twins

Like singletons, twins enter the formal school system in the preschool years ranging from the age of four to six in different societies. Preschool education is usually set up on a half day basis, consisting of morning or afternoon sessions. Like parents of singletons, parents of twins must choose which preschool they wish their twins to attend, but they must also decide whether they wish the twins to attend the same sessions or different sessions, morning versus afternoon or varying combinations of days of the week. For example, one goes Monday and Wednesday, the other goes Tuesday and Thursday, and they both go on Friday: the combinations come in multiples. If the twins do attend different sessions, the mother has the opportunity to spend time with each twin individually while the other twin is at preschool. This may be good for the twins and may help to encourage each twin's individuality, but it may also have some repercussions for the mother who has little time for herself. It may also result in some complications involving the scheduling of parental time in helping out in the preschool. But once the parental decision is made as to where and when the twins may go to preschool, the preschool has to be consulted and agree to take both of the twins and, hopefully, to take them as the parents so wish. While this sounds simple on paper, it does not always appear to be such an easy process in actual fact.

Most importantly, however, let's not lose sight of the fact that, if the decision is made to split the twins up in preschool, this is probably the first time that either twin has experienced such a lengthy separation. This would mean that the twins are required to interact with other children, with many twins engaging with others for the first time. The converse is also accurate: singletons may have to interact with twins for the first time and the former's reactions may deeply affect the latter.

Similar decisions have to be made when the twins are ready for **primary school**, including the issue of whether or not to separate the twins.

Let us assume that the parents have chosen the school - because of location, religious denomination, reputation - and the twins are eligible to attend and there are adequate places at this particular school. Some schools have educational policies which either insist on separating twins or insist on keeping them together in one class. Parental preference has little weight in some of these schools. On the other hand, some schools are willing or even anxious to consider the wishes of the parents, but they may or may not be in the relevant catchment area, the relevant religious denomination, and so on. Thus in some cases parents face a real dilemma about educating their twins even before the twins have entered an educational establishment - and more dilemmas usually follow.

Once in the school system, whether in the same class or **separated** into different classes, twins will deal with issues that singletons do not have to face. If they are separated for the first time, they may lose their sense of being twins, of being part of a unit. While many may consider that this is a positive process, it is still an added adjustment for the four- or five-year-old. On the other hand, if they are together in one classroom they may be treated as if they were one, treated as if they were not two individuals but rather were a unit. Their visibility may make them more susceptible to censure or blame ('the twins did it!') or more susceptible to suspicion of different forms of unacceptable behaviour ('the twins are talking!') While their behaviour may in fact be at the root of the to-be-specified problem, their visibility may make them more vulnerable or just more conspicuous children.

Another problem that twins face is that of **comparison.** In fact, comparison of and competition between the twins are the second most popular reasons given for separate placement of twins in school. Comparison may take the form of formal academic comparison in terms of conventional tests or national examinations. Or it may simply be related to which reading scheme each twin is working on. Parents who have experienced reading schemes which are designed not to let any child easily compare him/herself with other children's progress may be amazed at the lengths twins may go in order to determine who is reading the best or, to put it another way, which twin in winning the reading race! Scholastic comparison takes the form of grades, skills and other accomplishments, but it also colours which school the twin or twins will be able to attend when they transfer first to secondary school and later, perhaps, to university. Although twins are not necessarily equally endowed intellectually and may actually be markedly different in their intellectual ability, it is not hard to imagine some of the feelings and the problems faced by each twin in this situation. For example, the more successful twin might feel guilty (at the expense of his or her twin) as well as have feelings of accomplishment at being able to go to a 'better' school, and the other twin, when compared with his or her twin, might feel a failure.

Also significant in the school setting is athletic comparison: which twin is picked to play on which team? Is the same twin always chosen and is the same twin always left out or chosen last? The answer to this last question may be related to the area of socialising or **friendships**. One twin may, in fact, be more popular with school mates than his or her twin. One twin may have more friends and socialize more than the other. One twin may have a best friend and consequently the other twin is left out of this new relationship. For younger twins, problems often arise at classmates' birthdays and other socialising events. Parents of singletons may be concerned about inviting one twin without the other or may solve their concern by not inviting either twin. Many a (young) twin has needed consolation as the co-twin, by him or herself, is invited to and attends some special social event.

Back in the classroom, if the twins are not separated they -- unlike their singleton classmates -- are unable to be alone during the school day. They have no **privacy**. Neither one can come home and, in talking about their school day, fabricate or invent different events nor can they conceal other types of behaviour at school from the parents. In fact, the twin is unable to have or keep a secret from the parents as there is the other twin in the classroom. Another problem can occur with the **illness** of one twin. Here, in fact, is a chance for the healthy twin to be alone in the classroom, but he or she may find this a daunting prospect at first, especially if the twin relationship is a very dependent one.

Other factors affect twins in the school situation. Take **parents' evenings**. If the two children are in the same classroom, the teacher may simply lump the twins together and speak about 'the twins', evaluating them as if they were in fact a unit. Or the teacher may concentrate on a problem experienced by one twin at the expense of considering or discussing the progress of the other child. Other parents may also be frustrated and irritable about the time given to parents of twins, whether or not they know that the parents are parents of twins - 'Why are they taking so long - I thought we all had ten minutes!' The teacher of non-separated twins has been known to say, 'They are just the same. I can't tell them apart.' If, however, the children are in different classes, let alone different schools, other problems may arise, such as **scheduling** two distinct meetings with each teacher in primary school and with the many teachers in secondary school. Separate classes may also indicate that the problems one child may be having will not be considered when dealing with the other child: while it may not affect the other, it might be *a* or *the* vital factor or component. Of course Zoom meetings might ameliorate some problems!

The bottom line is one of identity. If the teacher on a parents evening is unable to differentiate the children adequately, how does this actually affect each twin daily in the classroom? And even if the twins are in separate classrooms, how do we excuse or condone the head teacher, who prides him or herself on knowing the names of every child in his or her school, asking one twin, *'Which one are you?'* The 'which one are you' factor is or may be a heavy consequence of twinship.

Death of a twin

This section could easily or equally have appeared previously where twinship is examined not from the twin(s)' point of view but from the perspective of other members in the family. Here both points of view will be discussed.

Let us start from a situation in which parents may face the possibility of the 'vanishing twin syndrome'. This syndrome refers to the loss of one of the twin foetuses in the womb, usually before the twelfth week of pregnancy. A twin pregnancy has been diagnosed by means of an ultrasound early in the pregnancy and at a later stage the 'twin' has vanished and is reabsorbed into the placenta. Parents of twins also face the possibility of early miscarriage, termination for foetal abnormality, the death of one of the twins in the womb between the twelfth and the twenty-eighth week of pregnancy (which are not recorded in the official birth figures), or even a still birth somewhat later on.

One twin may, however, die at birth or fairly soon thereafter. Any parent who loses a baby suffers a tragedy and parents of twins are no exception. But parents of twins have to cope with the loss of one child while at the same time coping with and caring for the other baby. In other words, they have to deal with birth and death simultaneously. How parents respond to their loss is a personal, individual and no doubt variable matter. Some Dutch research concludes that parents of twins who lose a twin at birth are likely to feel more anger and have stronger feelings of hostility than are the parents whose singleton dies at birth. Perhaps while this grief proceeds in the same order as for singletons, the intensity, duration and frequency -- depending on individual circumstances, age of gestation, type of loss, and, of course, the parents' backgrounds and modes of coping -- do differ.

Nonetheless, anger, resentment and guilt are feelings specified in all of the discussions about the loss of a twin child. The parent (in many cases especially the mother) also experiences a loss of pride, a loss of being special by dint of the very fact of having twins, as in 'Oh, here comes the mother of twins' in the labour ward before the birth. She then finds as she leaves the hospital with just one child, she goes unnoticed. However, she continues to regard herself as the mother of twins rather than the mother of a surviving singleton. 'There should have been two' is the phrase most often used by these mothers. How she and her partner simultaneously come to terms with the death of one twin and nurture the other twin is a moot point. Some mothers, for example, will overprotect the surviving twin. Others will blame and/or reject the surviving twin for the loss of the other child. Some will combine both reactions. Some will continue to favour or even begin to prefer the dead twin. Depending on gender, some will modify their treatment of the surviving twin. For example, if the boy dies, they may treat the girl as if she were a boy or perhaps treat her in a less favourable fashion. Some may even feel they only have half a baby.

The role of the **surviving twin** may thus be to act as a painful reminder of the loss of their twin or may equally act to comfort the parents for the loss of that twin. In fact, the very physical presence of the surviving twin in an identical pair is an especially visual, sometimes constant, reminder of the lost twin. For the surviving twin and the parents as well, anniversaries, such as birthdays, or traditional family holidays, such as Christmas, will be especially difficult times. And milestones in the surviving twin's life, such as starting school, being confirmed, going to university, or getting married, will most certainly be vivid reminders of the lost twin.

Parents need to grieve for the lost twin and take care of the surviving twin simultaneously, to whatever extent and in whatever way that is possible. Meanwhile, the surviving twin will be faced with the death of his or her twin and with coming to terms with this death. Obviously, the age at the time of the death of the twin sibling is an important variable in this process and the process will differ not only according to age but also from family to family and twin to twin.

It has been shown that the death of a twin -*at no matter what age* - is traumatic for the surviving twin. A very vivid example are 'singletons' who learn that they were actually born as twins but were raised as singletons. When made aware of their twin status, they may express a deep sense of loss and grief for that twin or a sense of unease about causing the death of the twin. Some may express satisfaction in completing an up-to-that time unsolved puzzle which had troubled them throughout their lives, feeling, that is, that there always was someone else.

Other twins lose their twin somewhat later on in life. Like their parents, they may experience anger and (unconscious) guilt over their twin's death, but in their case experience the guilt of being the survivor of the pair. Along with their feelings of profound loss and grief may be feelings of abandonment, loneliness, indecisiveness and uncertainty. The twin has lost not only a sibling, but has lost a twin sibling. Many suffer feelings of loss for many years which may increase as the twin gets older. The twin survivor must or may adapt to the death of their twin by means of a variety of adjustments. For example, some twins feel the need to talk to their absent twin. Some search for their twin in others or look for a replacement for their twin, sometimes in other relationships, sometimes in relation to their own children. Some twins name their own children after their lost twin. Some fear the isolation of being alone, of being a lone twin; some fear being themselves without their twin.

It could be argued that no one but a twin can actually understand or experience the immediate and long-term loss of the deceased twin. The need for a somewhat changed and/or changing identity for an individual who has been a twin since birth and has been recognized as part of a pair accompanies the death of a twin sibling. But no matter how labelled, the value of the twinship has been clearly diminished. The twin thus loses their twin through death which, in turn, equally upsets their place, their status, their very identity in the social world. Society more or less overlooks or takes little cognizance of the individual twin who loses a twin sibling.

ARE THEY IDENTICAL??

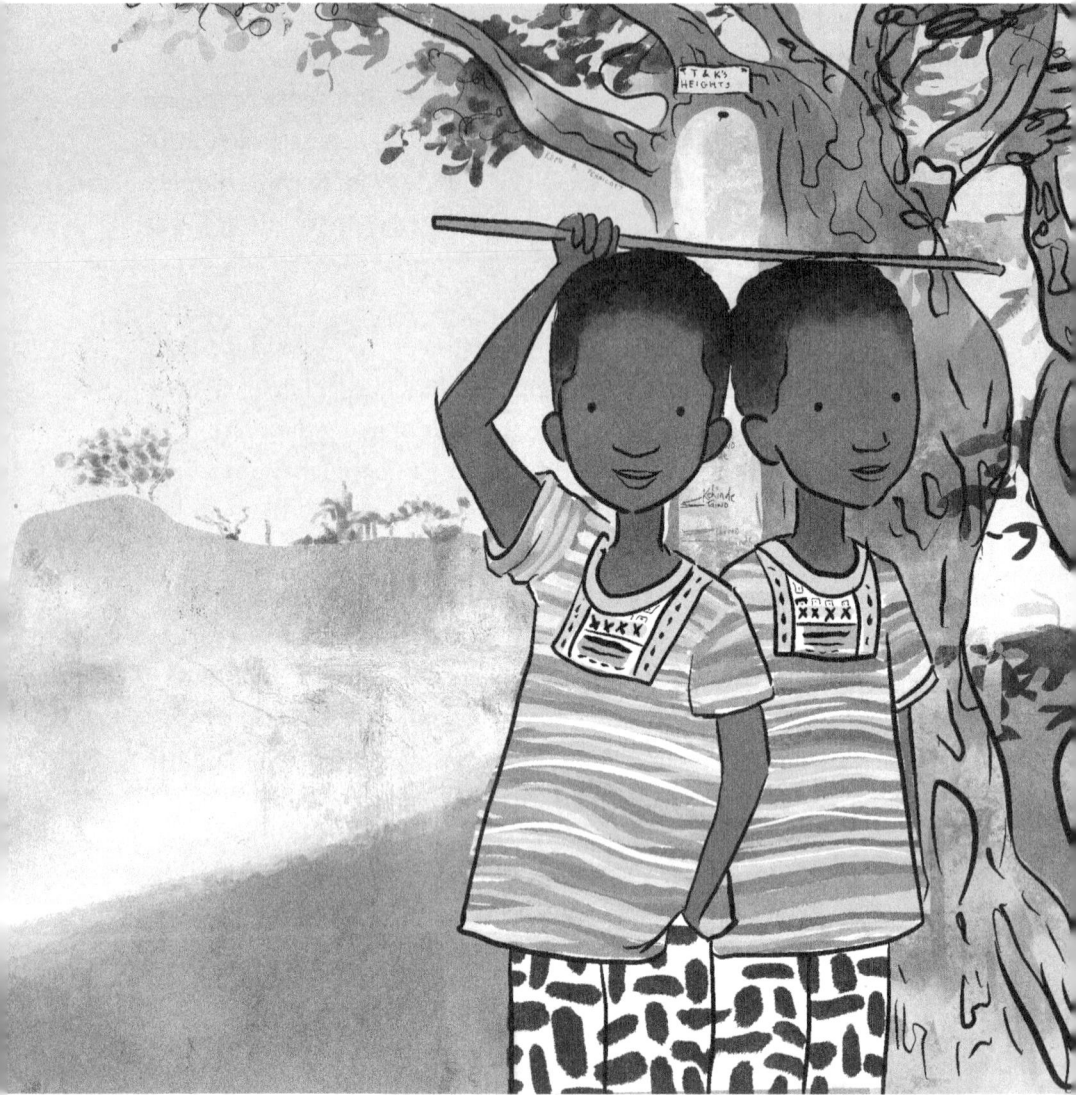

We've come this far and now let's look at the general public's reactions to twins. Research conducted in the UK discovered whether twins are seen in a positive or negative light and whether there is in fact any consensus on such views.

Many conferences and study days on aspects of twinship, largely organised in the UK by TAMBA (renamed Twins Trust), formed the base of the study. Interviewing mostly mothers of twins, the aim was to begin to find out British views about twins by asking the people who are at the forefront of such issues. The questionnaire was formalised into two questions which were administered to one hundred people at these conferences and study days over a period of three to four years. The overwhelming majority of people questioned were Caucasian, in the age range of twenty to forty. The participants were overwhelmingly parents of twins but in a few cases, respondents were related to people with twins, such as sisters or grandparents. Only eight were male. This was not a representative sample!

Parents of twins are uniquely placed to reflect on the reaction of others to the reality of twins. Most importantly, the parent respondents all more or less assumed that the interviewer did have twins herself, although this was confirmed only after the questionnaire was finished. This type of interviewer-as-participant approach allows the respondents to share the reactions they received from others in a quite relaxed - and eventually sharing - non-pressured manner. Parents of twins often share a unique bond and in my experience, a frank exchange of views is certainly made more possible because of this bond. In the course of trading experiences and exchanging anecdotes, some respondents answered in depth. Some reiterated their initial replies and emphasized certain aspects of their responses. This happened much more in the 'negative category' than in the 'positive category'.

It was predicted that the general reaction to twins would fall within the 'Aren't twins cute or adorable?' category. At the same time, it was imagined that, if the public would think that the idea of twins was more positive than negative, then their reactions would fall into the 'I wish *I were* a twin' category or 'Gee, I wish *I had* twins'.

The first question asked was: '**When you tell people you have twins, what is their reaction?**' While some replied only once to this question, others responded more fulsomely, thus explaining why the total number of responses - one hundred and ninety-eight - is greater than one hundred. Listed in descending order, the responses are as follows:

Table 9.1: Responses to first question: positive and negative

More positive responses:	Number
Lucky you, how nice, how lovely!	48
I've always wanted twins	18
Great!	12
You made a family all at once!	7
Aren't you clever to make two together!	6
What a surprise that must have been!	6
I'm a twin myself	5
Are there twins in your family?	4
I'll help you!	3
You must love being the centre of attention!	2
Total positive responses	111

The more negative responses were as follows:	Number
How do you cope?	36
What a burden (financial, physical, hands full)	28
Poor you!	11
Rather you than me!	4
I'd never manage	3
Double trouble	3
Was it a shock?	2
Total negative responses	87

The total number of positive responses was one hundred and eleven. The negative responses totalled eighty-seven, making twenty-four more positive than negative responses. More respondents answered twice in the positive than in the negative categories. Moreover, of those who responded only once in the negative, their replies tended to be most emphatic. For example, the four who answered, 'Rather you than me' were very aware of other people's reactions to their twins, so much so that the phrase 'rather you than me ' was repeated with great feeling and a certain knowing look, specifically indicating that the phrase 'rather you than me' actually meant '*better* you than me'.

Forty-two respondents gave both positive and negative responses. For example, a woman with nineteen-month-old boy twins said that people reacted to her twins by saying 'Oh, how lovely! How do you cope?' A woman with two-and-a-half-year-old boy twins responded, 'They say, I've always wanted twins, but my, don't you have your hands full!' So of the more than forty per cent of respondents who answered in both positive and negative categories, one might feel that they were actually attempting to demonstrate two not altogether incompatible reactions. In other words, an initial negative response may have been followed by a more positive response (such as in 'What a burden that must be! but 'Great, you made a family all at once!') given that some of the general public *might have* been aware of the delicacy of the matter. On the other hand, a more positive response could easily have led to a more 'realistic' response, as in the instance of 'What a surprise that must have been!' followed by 'I'd never manage.'

The second question asked of all the respondents was: **'Once people knew you had twins, what was their first question to you?'** The responses were, in ascending numerical order:

Table 9.2: Responses to 'Once people knew you had twins, what was their first question to you?

Are they as alike as two peas in a pod?	1
When did you find out about having twins?	2
Who was born first/ second?	4
Temperament: who dominates, how do they get on?	6
What gender are they?	9
Are they identical?	84
Total	106

The first obvious point to be made is that the range of answers to this question is very limited indeed. Starting with the least popular answer -- 'Are they as alike as two peas in a pod?' -- we note that much twin research uses this phrase when asking parents or teachers or whomever to distinguish identical twins from fraternal twins. However, only one respondent out of the one hundred answered by using the pea pod analogy. The next three answers are certainly questions specific to having twins: when did you discover that you were having twins; what was the birth order of your twins (who was first and who was second); and what sort of temperament do they have in relation to each other? This last question involved comments such as how do the twins get on together and which one is the leader. One mother volunteered that she was asked who was the *good* twin. The second most numerous question asked was about the gender of the twins, but that question could equally have applied to the birth of any child, whether it be a single birth or multiple birth child. However, the question overwhelmingly asked of parents of twins was, 'Are they identical?'. Almost every parent cited this response.

Discussion

In general, judging from the first part of the parents of twins questionnaire, the public's attitude towards twins is somewhat more positive than negative. The largest category of responses contained the reply 'Lucky you, how nice, how lovely!' to the fact of the twins. However, while some parents reported that this was indeed the responses they received, other parents indicated that the public continued by asking more probing questions, such as 'How do you cope?' and 'What a burden they must be!' Only one respondent indicated that the response to her twins varied with age, that is, people in the older age group who were no longer in the childbearing age saw the twins as cute, lucky, very positive. Those in the childbearing group were more concerned with the practicalities of actually parenting twins and all that that involved.

Without any doubt, almost all of the respondents, that is, eighty four per cent, answered the second part of the questionnaire with the question most asked of them, namely, '**Are your twins identical?** ' The respondents themselves concluded that once the public learned about the presence of twins, their first reaction or assumption was that twins by their very nature *were* identical. Even those parents of boy/girl twins were constantly asked if their twins were identical! One father reports that, having told people about his boy/girl twins, he was still asked, 'Aren't they *a bit* identical then?' And parents of obviously non-identical twins (for example, those parents whose twins had very different hair colouring as young children) were also asked if indeed their twins were not identical.

Almost all of the respondents replied only once to this question, and they did so almost in a chant or a mantra or mockingly repeating, 'Are they identical?' Of the very few parents who responded twice to this question, only one person did not include the answer about twins being identical. There was virtually no hesitation in the response to the question. In other words, the conclusion drawn from this part of the project is that the perceived or assumed identical nature of twinship concerned or interested people most.

This project reveals current attitudes towards twins in our culture. Although we know that twins are distinctive or different from singletons, it appears that our first reaction is to enquire whether or not they are 'identical'. The basic assumption seems to be that twins are -- or, as some argued, *should* be – identical. Twinship by its very nature involves two individuals who are the same, who look alike, who wear the same clothes. The association of similarity or 'identicalness' with the word twins, as well as the images of twins being largely appearance based, was revealed. Also uncovered was the fact that images of twins fell within the area of babies or children as our associations with doubleness are child-oriented.

The second conclusion is that the scales tip in favour of the view of twinship as being slightly more positive. This strongly supports the view of twinship as perhaps the idealised or fantasised view of twinship. This sees twins not only as 'identical' but also as uniquely close people who are lucky enough to have a best friend.

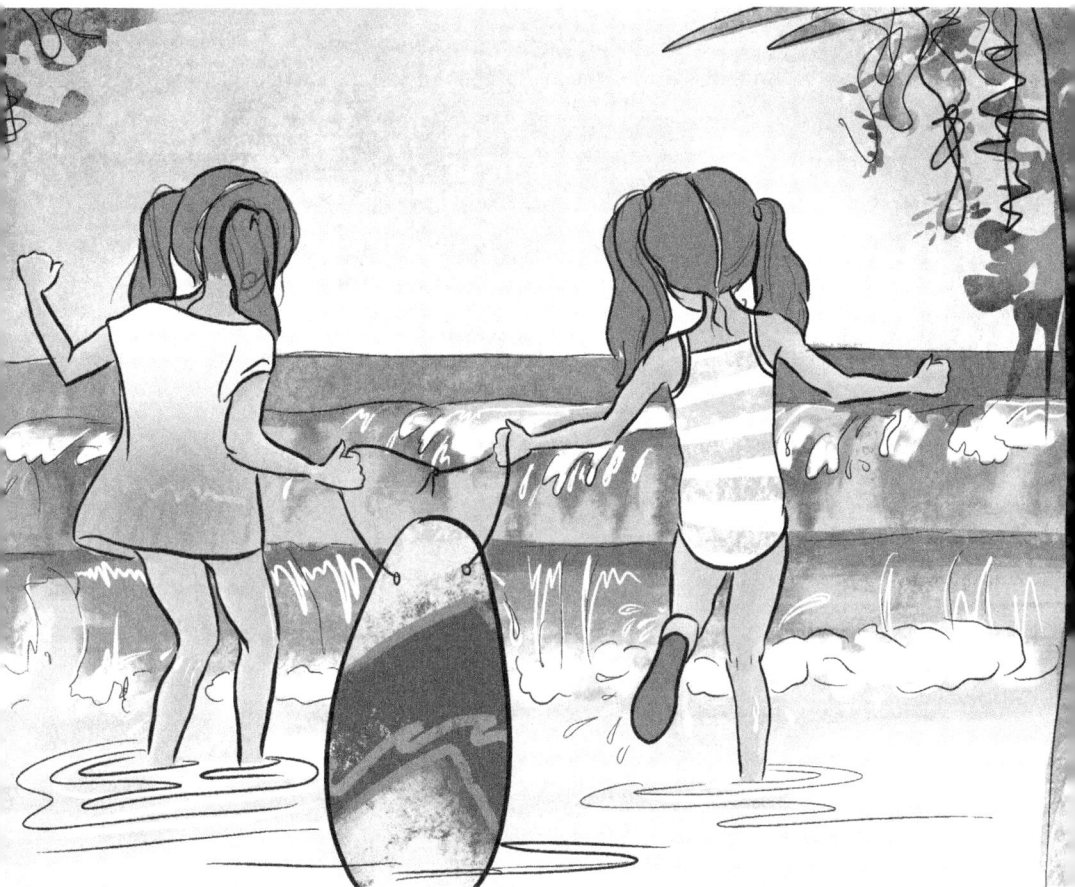

S ome twins, especially identical females, grow up in social surroundings which recognise and expect the twins to be, to act, to become and to be treated as very similar to each other. Pressure to conform in childhood is considerable. Other sets of twins, brought up in families who are consciously trying to help their twins to individualise, are equally expected NOT to be so similar.

However, as both groups are in fact twins, each twin within the pair may experience tension when the role of 'twin' conflicts with other roles that they may wish to play. For example, each one may wish to be *the best* basketball player or *the prettiest* girl at the dance or to be simply siblings rather than a 'twin' brother or 'twin' sister. This type of tension usually changes with time, age and circumstances. For some twins, twinship is a chronic but not necessarily intense embarrassment. 'He's not really my twin brother!' or 'Do we always have to go to swimming together?' For other twins, their wish to have been born as singletons is overwhelming and helps to determine or at least significantly condition their behaviour. For still others, twinship is worn as an exceedingly proud stigma, even as a badge: 'My sister and I, we're twins, you know. We're inseparable; we were born with a best friend!'

Cannot a twin choose whether or not to be a twin? For example, when a twin goes separately to university, he or she may not mention his or her twinship. Different contexts at different stages of life may lead the individual twin to present different selves so that the reaction to twinship may range from acceptance to rejection or vice versa. Some twins conceal the twinship and portray themselves as a singleton. Another way the twin attempts to reduce tension – some would say, attention – is by hiding or modifying the twinship. In some cases, a confidante could be selected who would know the 'real' truth about the identity of the twin. Some twins manipulate the environment or the situation as they define it and then adopt strategies which result from this. The phenomenon of 'double trouble' or other behavioural problems especially found in the classroom where both twins are kept together are often the outcomes. On the other hand, there are both amusing and not so amusing stories of identical and/or fraternal twins taking the place of their same-sex twins - in the classroom, on a date or at a job interview.

As we have already seen, stereotypes of twinship are transmitted in the press, in films, and in television commercials. The *identical* nature of twinship is implied and acknowledged. We tend to stereotype all twins as identical and assume that they are identical. These simplifications, generalisations and assumptions have sometimes helped to inhibit the individual development of some twins, that is, the development of twins *as* individuals.

Stereotypes about twins are also based on the idea that twinship involves an emotionally close relationship between the pair, especially between same-sex twins. This assumes that each twin's needs and feelings are automatically met and understood by the other twin. The assumed (or stereotyped) closeness of the twins may subsequently have serious consequences. Some twins do indeed internalise these expectations and become anxious and confused by the very fact that they do not conform to the stereotype and do not experience this intimacy. In these cases, some fight constantly with their twin and, at times, regard their twin as their bitterest rival.

The stereotype of emotional closeness is also assumed to indicate a shared identify, a unit identity. The two individuals are treated as one unit, as a 'we' rather than an 'I' plus (or minus) another 'I'. This unit identity may take the form of, 'Let me introduce you to the twins or to the Smith twins' rather than 'Let me introduce you to Stephanie and Gwendolyn'. Stephanie and Gwendolyn also hear themselves linked together in 'Stephanie and Gwendolyn Smith' whereas other children may hear Stephanie Smith and Gwendolyn Smith. Twins may respond to this joint introduction by saying, 'I am not "the twins": I have my own name!'

Twins are often lumped together when they are labelled as twins and treated not as two individuals but as one. But this labelling could also be specifically applied *between* the twins themselves. One variable would be what consequences flow from identifying and treating one twin as the elder and one twin as the younger: 'How I have suffered because she was always the boss' says the younger girl twin by ten minutes. Or in other families, the elder twin is accorded a variety of privileges denied to the younger. Another variable relates to splitting the twin unit into opposites, whereby one twin is labelled the 'good' twin and the other the 'bad' twin. The labels 'good' and 'bad', which accentuate similarities as well as differences in a twin pair, could be applied equally to various character traits. These could include sociability or shyness, athletic prowess (he who excels in sport and she who can't hit a ball), physical attributes (fat or thin, or more fat and less thin, or pretty and prettier), and intellectual or academic ability. Achievement in the school system also helps in this process with the emphasis here on bright and not so bright.

A final label relates to the nature of twinship. The question is often asked of twins, 'Are you identical?' to which some may then add, 'Or are you fraternal?' The label of identical twin or fraternal twin for many twins themselves spells confusion. This is not only dependent on the age of the twin but on the fact that some twins do not actually know whether or not they are indeed monozygotic (identical) or dizygotic (fraternal) twins. But in either instance, what does either label mean? Does 'identical' merely refer to genetic similarity or does it have more far-reaching consequences?

While it seems that our mental picture of twins falls primarily within the 'Are they identical?' mode, it seems possible that our conceptions may be modified by the very fact that medical procedures such as IVF and scientific research into the development of the cloning of animals are being more frequently aired in public. This is linked to the fact that more and more twins are now born, as confirmed by the increase in the birth rate of twins and higher multiples.

Twins as a minority group??

In certain respects, twins are a distinctive group - a minority group - who may in fact face differences and/or disadvantages which are related to twinship. Twins are singled out as being special. They are widely noticed and receive attention for their twinship. Their distinctiveness may provoke a variety of reactions which may lead to their own confusion: not only are they known as the twins or as Stephanie and Gwendolyn, but 'I, Gwendolyn, know (or I think I know) that I am Gwendolyn, so why are you calling me Stephanie? Does anybody know *me*?' At the other end of this spectrum is: 'Are you, Stephanie and Gwendolyn, really twins? You *don't look like* twins.' These reactions may all be eliminated when at a certain age twins (may) split up and lead more separate lives, although it is not hard to think of the confusion experienced by fellow workers, let us say, when a twin's twin appears unannounced alongside the originally known twin.

In general when we become pregnant, we expect to have one child and this 'one' child may be maintained by treating twins as one and the same. We tend to relate to and treat twins 1) as a unit, as two halves of a divided whole in which one-half plus one-half makes only one twinship or 2) as two copies of the same individual in which one twin and his or her co-twin equal only one twin copy. In both cases, twins are two but are treated as one. As some twins say, here is 'my other half' or we 'live life as one person' or 'we are the same because neither of us wants one to be better than the other!'

Identity formation or Who Am I?

Finally or in the very beginning, the relationship with the mother is different for twins. Each twin must share the mother with the co-twin from the very beginning. This fact of sharing, argue most researchers, interferes with or - at the very least - alters the maternal relationship. It follows therefore that the bottom line in identity formation in twins is different from identity formation in singletons.

So each twin faces a complex task of becoming an individual. In some twin pairs, the twinship may be instrumental in providing the impetus needed to differentiate between the twins, each on his/her separate path towards self-development. In order to be 'me', I must be different from my co-twin. The tension between a growing sense of one's identity and increasing pressures for rebelling, as well as for social conformity, are additional pressures. If both twins rebel in the same direction, are they rebelling or conforming? Who goes in which direction and is it a conscious move? And if twins share the same friends, how do they distinguish themselves - from the friends, from the co-twin? This process of differentiation may be lengthy and painful, but may avoid other feelings which may arise from the twins' distinctive achievements and other rivalries, as well as from relationships with others. In developing an identity, then, twins do so in relation not only to the parent(s) but also specifically in relation to the co-twin.

Unlike twins, the rest of us are not confronted with sweeping statements about our *lack of individuality*. Many geneticists say that everybody is different or unique, except for identical twins. And some go so far as to say that twins are perfect copies of each other - they are clones. Not in my mind, however.

CONCLUDING REMARKS

I n all known societies, twins occupy a special place. From myths, through drama and literature to social science research, the fantasies and realities of twinship have continued to provide an endless source of fascination, pleasure and disturbance. In general, traditional societies fear twins as 'unnatural', whereas modern or postmodern-societies are generally more accepting of the 'unusual'. At the same time, modern societies also place twins at the centre of an insoluble dilemma. The dilemma is each twin's need to internalise or at least inhabit individual roles, thereby minimising the significance of being a twin, while at the same time being chronically confronted with a role which above all prioritises the fact of being a twin.

What both types of societies share in common is that when a woman says she is 'expecting', it is assumed that she is expecting one child. Single births are the norm, *the* reference point. Children/babies are literally and invariably measured in relation to singletons, measured in terms of weight, growth, developmental landmarks, etc. To a very large extent, from conception through gestation, childbirth and subsequently into childhood and adolescence, people are measured in *unitary terms*. Twins are an anomaly to such processes, creating the very paradoxes illuminated throughout this book.

The critical question which remains is whether there are specific factors which apply only to the twin situation. The answer would appear to be a qualified *yes* if we accept the following:

1) the ***biological factors*** of twinship, which may determine intrauterine and perinatal risks for and outcomes to each or both of the twins;

2) the fact of a ***triadic*** rather than (or even in addition to) a dyadic ***relation*** between mother and two infants;

3) the **psychoanalytic** principles /thoughts about the nature and consequences of the twin relationship or twin bond; and

4) the very essence of the **social nature** of twinship itself, namely, the **presence of two** people who, especially in childhood, are not only developing in the company of and interacting with each other, but also face their social world together, (relationally) linked.

In essence, twins are different, distinct, special. As we have seen, for example, a great deal of effort is required for twin childcare in relation to finance, time, emotional and psychic energy. Only the parents of twins know the specific and in some ways insoluble dilemmas involved. Similarly, only twins themselves know what it is actually like to be a twin - although, as a corollary, they do not know what it is like to be a singleton. Finally, in contemporary societies, it is certainly the case that enquiries about twins, whether unborn or existing, almost invariably take the form, 'Are they identical?' The accompanying unspoken assumption, hope or even' knowledge', is that the answer is 'yes'. To the extent that postmodern culture prioritises individuality and difference, twinship requires us to reflect upon an irreducible social bond.

In the end, only a twin really knows the joys, the fun and the pitfalls of being a twin! Hoorah for them!!

Further Reading

Abbink, C. et al 'Bonding as perceived by mothers of twins', *Paediatric Nursing*,8 (1982), 411-13.

Bryan, E.M. *The Nature and Nurture of Twins*. London: Bailliere Tindall, 1983.

Burlingham, D. *Twins – A Study of Three Paiars of Identical Twins*. New York: International Press, 1952.

Cooper, C. *Twins and Multiple Births: the essential Parenting Guid from Pregnancy to Adulthood*. London: Vermillion, 1997.

Cronin, H.J. 'An analysis of the neuroses of identical twins', *Psychoanalytic Review*, 20 (1933); 375-87

Davis, D.L. *Twins Talk: What Twins Tell us about Person, Self and Society*. Athens, OH: Ohio University Press, 2014.

deBres, H. *How to be Multiple*. Manchester: Manchester University Press, 2024.

Friedman, J.A. *Emotionally healthy Twins*. Cambridge, Ma: DaCapo Press, 2008.

Friedman, J. A. The *Same but Different*. Los Angeles, Ca: Rocky Pines Press, 2013.

Gedda, L. *Twins in History and Science*. Springfield, IL: Charles C. Thomas, 1961.

Hartmann, H. *Essays on Ego Psychology*. London: the Hogarth Press and the Institute of Psycho-Analysis, 1964.

Harvey, D. and Bryan, E. (eds) *The Stress of Multiple Births*. Hereford, UK: Multiple Births Foundation, 1991.

Hay, D.A. et al. 'The older sibling of twins', *Australian Journal of Early Childhood*, 13 (19988): 25-8.

Karpman, B. 'Psychodynamics in fraternal twinship relations', *Psychoanalytic Review*, 40 (1953): 243-67.

LaRossa, R. *Becoming a Parent*. London: Sage, 1986.

Leonard, M. 'Twins: the myth and the reality', *Child Study*,30 (1953): 9-13.

Leonard, M. 'Problems in identification and ego development in twins', *Psychoanalytic Study of the Child*, 16 (1961): 300-20.

Linney, J. 'The emotional and social aspects of having twins', *Nursing Times*,76 (1981): 276-9.

Linney, J. *Multiple Births*. Chichester: Wiley and Sons, 1983.

Mahler, M.S et al. *The Psychological Birth of the Human Infant*. New York: Basic Books, 1975.

Peek, P.M. ed. *Twins in African and Diaspora Cultures: Double Trouble, Twice Blessed*. Bloomington, In, Indiana University Press,2011. ???

Piontelli, A. *Twins in the World*. New York: Palgrave Macmillan, 2008.

Robarge, J.P. et al.'Increased child abuse in families with twins', *Researching in Nursing and Health*, 5 (1982): 199-203.

Rosembeau, M. *How Twins Grow Up*. London: Bodley Head, 1987.

Sandbank, A. *Twins and the family*. Guilford, Surrey: TAMBA, 1988.

Segal, N. *Entwined Lived: Twins and what they tell us about Human Behaviour*. New York: Dutton Press, 1999.

Showers, J et al #Research in twins: implications for parenting', *Child: Care, Health and Development*, 10(6) (1984): 391-404.

Stewart, E.A. *Exploring Twins: towards a social analysis of twinship*. London: Palgrave Macmillan, 2003.

Stewart, E.A. *Twin Tales: Hand in Hand across the World* KDP, Amazon, 2020.

Taylor, E.M. et al 'Maternal stress, family and health care of twins', *Children and Society,* 2(4) (1988-9): 351-19.

Wallace, M. *The Silent Twins*. London: Chatto and Windus, 1986.

Winnicott, DW. *The Child, the Family and the Outside World*. London: Penguin, 1991.

Woodward, J. *The Lone Twin: Understanding Twin Bereavement and Loss*. London: Free Association Books, 1998.

Wright, L. *Twins: Genes, Environment and the Mystery of Human Identity*. London: Weidenfeld and Nicolson, 1997.

Text: Dr Elizabeth A. Stewart, 2024

Illustrations: Kemi Athene Pennicott

Moral rights asserted

Also by the author:

Exploring Twins: towards a social analysis of twinship,

Twin Tales: Hand in Hand across the World,

and

From Russia with Hope: Russian Women's

Journeys to the West

Contact: dr_eastewart@hotmail.co.uk

Printed in Great Britain
by Amazon